Forge

Helen Morrell

chipmunk ~~publishing~~
the mental

Helen Morrell

Published by
Chipmunkapublishing
PO Box 6872
Brentwood
Essex CM13 1ZT
United Kingdom

http://www.chipmunkapublishing.com

Edited by Aleks Lech

Chipmunkapublishing gratefully acknowledge the support of Arts Council England.

The History and Development of Mill House and Community Support Homes

1984	April	Dave, Helen and two sons, Shane (aged 9) and Lee (aged 7) moved into Mill House, Gayton
1984	June	First unofficial resident
1985	Oct	Registered with Homes Registration
1989	July	No. 14 Portland Street opened. Small residential home in town of King's Lynn
1990	July	Third son, Jake born
1992	April	Fourth son, Charlie born
1993	May	Purchased 2 Mill Cottage on the Gayton site for three residents to live independently
1993	June	Family moved out of Mill House into the bungalow a few minutes walk away in Gayton
1995		Lynwood Terrace opened. Property in King's Lynn for semi-independent residents
1996	Oct	Adrian Lodge opened. Small residential Home in King's Lynn/Houses became more know as Community Support Homes
1998		No 2, Archdale Street opened. Units for semi-independent residents in King's Lynn
1999		No. 12, Portland Street opened. Small residential home

2002 Dec Purchased 1 Mill Cottage. Live in by supported married couple plus office space for Business Manager

2007 July Dave and Helen retired

The purpose of Mill House and Community Support Homes was to offer short-term, emergency care as an alternative to hospital as well as semi-independent bedsits and shared accommodation within the main houses or in close proximity to one of them. By 2007, the 10 units could hold up to 53 residents.

INTRODUCTION

Hi, I'm Helen. For twenty five years myself, my partner and four sons have had the privilege to live and work alongside people suffering with and recovering from mental illness in our rambling grade two listed building in the heart of the Norfolk countryside. Little did we realize when we embarked on this venture what a roller coaster journey it would be. We were clueless in our ideals and naïve as to what was to come in our residential care home.

We opened up Mill House first and as time went by the business developed from being just the Mill House to including three more residential care homes and two supported housing units. As experience grew so the thinking, philosophy and practices of Community Support Homes developed and took shape.

What I would like to achieve from this book is for you to have some understanding of the issues relating to mental health which I have perhaps learnt in a non conventional way during my very exciting years working closely with some very 'colourful characters'. I have been determined to remain honest to, and about, myself, 'warts' and all. It is so important for people to be seen as individuals. I am grateful for being blessed with an abundance of energy and drive which I have channeled into a love of my working life.

I hope I will manage to share with you the good times, bad times and humorous times from the past twenty five years. I have strived passionately to reduce the stigma attached to mental health. I have throughout my working life, at times, tried to take on 'the system' when it has failed troubled individuals.

So many people have contributed to this book. They have been social workers, professional carers, residents, parents and my friends and family. Some people have dearly wanted to contribute but found revisiting their past too painful. I have deeply respected that. For those who have contributed I feel it has at times been helpful to them and to myself. My aim is to share their experiences so that their stories can be heard.

CHAPTER ONE

I was born Helen Easton and have one sister and two brothers. My parents were very supportive to us and ran their own businesses. My dad was a self employed coal merchant and my mother ran her own newsagents shop. There were times when my mum would be in the yard with my dad bagging up coal by floodlight late into the night!

I remember when I was about four I used to deliver papers for my mum, as all the family had to have a paper round. I delivered to a couple of chaps called George and Bill Curson who lived across the road from us. They had lost their mother, neither of them had married and they lived in this little stone cottage which had no kitchen but only a corrugated iron lean-to with one little electric burner to cook on. They always made me so welcome there. They lived in squalor to be honest, and they certainly didn't have a cleaner, not seeing cleaning as a priority. For instance, George used to keep a spittoon next to his chair and nearly always had what I can only describe as a grubby hand rolled cigarette stuck to his bottom lip. As I got older I used to go and help them out a bit and they used to give me Quality Street. I would do things like fry them eggs on a Saturday morning. I loved their quaint loo which was a bucket with a big wooden seat on it in a shed outside. This loo required pumping out weekly which was not for the faint hearted. I remember there were lots of birds nesting in the roof of the shed and it was quite exciting to sit there and watch the birds go to and fro. Unbeknown to me I think my time spent with these two gentlemen formed the foundations of my interest in wanting to care for people.

In my early teenage years I used to go out selling firelighters for my dad which was a good grounding in meeting and negotiating with people. These firelighters were a job lot that he had found and were perhaps past their sell by date and so virtually 'unlightable'; as one of my customers pointed out, "it took me almost a whole box of matches to light it."

I had wanted a pony for about as long as I could walk and talk. My parents went to Watton horse sale and came home with a beautiful hot-headed 12.2 hands four year old. I was ten years old and had no riding experience other than my metal framed rocking horse and a few rides on my friend's horse up the road. It was the most inappropriate purchase, but my dad loved a bargain, and this glossy coated liver chestnut had taken his eye as a good buy. Neither of my parents had the slightest idea of what suitable meant. My mother was terrified of the creatures. The pony was called Johnny and the love I had for him gave me grit and determination for the future. On one occasion Johnny galloped with me flat out along the A47, an immensely busy road that claims many drivers' lives, let alone the life of a child fiercely clinging to the pommel of a crazy pony. Johnny galloped the last two miles home with me clinging on for dear life.

Due to my non-existent experience with horses he was allowed to be outrageously naughty at times. For instance, he dragged me around a field hung from a stirrup by one foot until the leather gave way and I bounced onto the wet grass...
It was not unusual for him to run out of control with me desperately trying to pull him up.

On another occasion he somersaulted me into a ditch where he became stuck in the mud until rescued by a local farmer who had witnessed the incident from his bedroom window. He hauled him out with a rope attached to his truck. This incident occurred because we had been racing another horse, failed to negotiate a corner and discovered too late that a large ditch was too wide to jump. On reflection I think this was one of many examples when I have been looked after by a 'Guardian Angel'.
I continued to be deeply involved with horses and in my early teens used to take part in competitive eventing on behalf of a Canadian family who owned a large string of horses. I was fearless and would take on challenges most other people would avoid. One of my jobs was to return the horses from a field to the stables, and I would jump the two five bar gates with only the head collar on the horse but no protective hat or saddle.

I went on to Secondary school and by then I was a rebel determined to be thrown out. I was completely headstrong and was seen as a pain by the teachers. Despite being a show off and often totally inappropriate in school I did lack confidence. I think this later enabled me to empathize with people who had little confidence.

By the age of sixteen I had left school with a handful of CSEs, was pregnant and was soon married! I think this was when I realized how determined I can be, because it didn't even occur to me that I might not cope. I worked at a livery yard and would take my son, Shane, with me. As soon as he could sit up I used to go out riding, with him on the front of the saddle. My second son Lee was born eighteen months later and what another wonderful character he was. At this time I did less at the stables and took on voluntary work at an incredibly vibrant youth club. We used to go camping and facilitate activity groups, summer holidays, canoeing and just about anything you can think of. I've always had a fantastic amount of energy so it suited me well. I probably wasn't the most responsible mum and Lee got lost on one occasion after being carried off by some girls to play, but no harm came to him. He had just wandered off and dropped off to sleep under the Youth and Community Officer's desk!

I later returned to education via the local college and obtained a variety of qualifications.
I was happily married for eight years but circumstances changed and to be honest I outgrew my husband. I left my marriage and eventually became good friends with Dave Morrell which influenced my decision to move on with my life in a different direction. I had moved in with my Aunt Bet who was one of my most favourite people ever. She lived in South Lynn and she always said her door was open to me if ever I wanted to leave because at times she knew I was not overly happy where I was. So I left my very comfortable three bed roomed bungalow and moved in with Aunt Bet, obviously taking Shane who was six years old and Lee, four years old, with me.

I left my husband on a Thursday and went to a Jumble sale the following Saturday and collected up lots of second hand clothes as I thought I had better earn some money quickly, not having any regular income apart from my family allowance which I had agreed to give to my aunt each week. I collected bags of jumble, offered £1 for each bag, bought a clothes rail for 25p and had two pasting tables with an old carry cot that I bought for 50p.

I set off for the market with my Citroen Dyane stuffed to the gunnels with all my goodies that I bought from the jumble sales on Saturday, to earn a few quid. It was exciting to explore my new found independence. Existing stallholders frowned upon me really because my stall looked a bit of a shambles. People looked upon my stall as an unruly untidy load of junk arriving next to them and detracting from their smart stalls. This was the era before car boot sales existed. The market superintendent and I got on very well and I would chat him up to get a pitch because in those days there was very little space for casual workers. I had to drop my boys off at school before I could get round to the market and so I was never one of the 'early birds' either. Very often he would say that the whole market was full but I would walk round and find a little nook or cranny with just enough space for a table with a little rail squashed in as well. I became well known on the market and I loved it. It was really enjoyable and on a good day's takings we would have some good food or buy something nice. Sometimes I was so skint I couldn't afford to put petrol in the car and had to put both boys on my bike from South Lynn and wheel them up together to the school which was really quite a haul. Things were a bit tight but nevertheless I was happy. Auntie always offered warmth and comfort, she was great. After leaving my marriage my relationship with Dave blossomed and we had a friendship for some time. By now he had left his wife because he was unhappy and living in rented accommodation in an old farmhouse in Stanfield.

About six months after I had moved in with Aunt I received a phone call to say that George Curson had died. I hadn't kept regular contact with him but I always used to make an effort if I visited Mum and Dad who lived opposite to him and I would stick my head in to say hello. Anyway, just before George died in hospital after Christmas, Dad and I went up to see him to take him a present. We took him some slippers because he had absolutely nobody to care about him. I enjoyed having a chat with the old boy really, and you know it gives you a good feeling looking out for someone who hasn't got much.

But then something sad but wonderful happened. There was a phone call from a solicitor saying that George Curson had died and that he had left his house to me! So the paper girl gets left a cottage, like something out of a Mills and Boon story! However the biggest surprise was that the property they left me, which I was able to sell for £18,000, gave Dave and me the opportunity of moving in together and buying our own home.

On one of my visits to George's house as a teenager, he gave me a locket with a picture of his mother inside. Years later the locket became very significant. On the front it said 'Forget Me Not'. I've often wondered if this is when he made his will. I will never know. Were they very pertinent words for characters I would later work with? I only wish he could look down and see what leaving his house to me achieved and how it enabled me to help and guide many people through difficult times.

That was twenty six years ago.

Dave and I wanted to create our own business in the caring profession. I was always a good cook and housekeeper and I had a zest for life, initiative and common sense. Dave was a Divisional Youth and Community Officer and a Social Worker. I always thought he would be our "front man" and do the 'professional bits', admin and organization etc., and I would take on the cooking, cleaning and housekeeping side. We didn't have a clue about where to start, so we set about exploring ideas. Our first step was to get some money together and we purchased our first property in Foulsham. It was a complete wreck which had a closure order on it. It had no bathroom and only a well outside which you had to pump water from. When a builder visited to

11

give an estimate for the work that needed to be done, he fell through from the first floor into the kitchen in front of us, so that gives you some idea what state the place was in! Anyway, we decided this was for us, the aim being if we worked on the renovation of this property, we would earn some money to put towards our future dream of running our own business in the caring profession. I got a cleaning job a few doors up with a rich London guy who had his own house in Wimbledon and who was luckily away during the week. I used to cheekily hop into the shower periodically to have a scrub up because it was just filthy in our house, and I used their loo because they had a flushable toilet. Our house was a small part of a big Victorian house and the big part was owned by some very "upper crust" people who really thought the gypsies had arrived and moved in next door. Due to the renovating work which went on for a number of months we had no bathroom and had to use a chemical loo. Dave used to go into the garden and dig a big hole where he would empty it, but in severe weather when there was frost this became impossible.   This meant we constantly had to assess whether there was any room left in it for just one more wee. This is where my cleaning job came in handy with their real toilet!

One of my work duties was to clean out the fridge where there were all sorts of wonderful things to eat. There used to be rare roast beef, half a salmon and my instructions were – "Helen, could you please clean out the fridge and dispose of the contents" so I did! Being a complete gannet I used to cut off great big chunks of the beef and eat them there and then. On one particular day I was very lucky because a situation arose that could have been terribly embarrassing. I'd been in the downstairs shower, I'd gone through to the kitchen, I had gorged on leftovers in the fridge and after feeling much cleaner and fresher and with a full belly I headed off up the stairs with my cleaning cloths and various other bits and pieces.

I walked into the master bedroom and nearly jumped out of my skin because, peering out of those beautiful bed covers, was a little blond headed, skinny faced, gay chap. The owner of the house was gay and he had brought one of his London boyfriends home with him but hadn't informed me. He was well spoken and after being disturbed by me almost jumped out of his skin. After apologising, he bid me good morning but I was quite grateful that he hadn't come down to see me sitting on the loo or naked in the shower.

There was no Nouvelle Cuisine in our kitchen, as we only had a small gas burner. However, I would create some interesting concoctions for the family meals. In addition to this there were frequent visits to the chip shop. We did a lot of the work ourselves alongside the builder, which was great fun, but we also took time out to play hours of football with children from the village, using makeshift goals in the field at the back of our property. I also met a wonderful woman called Victoria and she used to let me ride her horse. Life was good and we were all very happy.

I continued doing market stalls because that used to bring in some good income whilst Dave continued working in Norwich as a social worker, and slowly we developed this house into a very pretty cottage. Once we completed the cottage we decided we would put it up for sale and put an advert in the Sunday Times. The first people who rang eventually bought the property. Unfortunately, I had a little calamity before they arrived. We were working on our plan to try and find a suitable property for our own business to run as a residential home of some sort. A friend of mine called round to help me consider a number of properties that I had details of around the Kings Lynn area. I forgot that I had put a chip pan on for dinner and our dog Lucy kept barking at the kitchen door. I kept saying "oh be quite Lucy", until smoke started seeping under the door of the utility room. I opened the door and the kitchen was on fire and we quickly evacuated the house! By sheer chance we lived next door to a garage and a very brave, or very silly, passer by ran to the garage, grabbed a fire extinguisher, and attacked the fire which by that time was raging with swirling black smoke pouring from the windows. He had almost put it out by the time the fire brigade arrived. It was very sad because we had worked so hard on the property.

We were expecting prospective buyers at that time so I phoned them and said that unfortunately we had been called away on important business and that they wouldn't be able to come for a week because I didn't want to tell them the kitchen had been on fire! There were melted buttons on the hob but perhaps they wouldn't notice! In fact, even the week after, we were still not ready for them and had to put them off for a few more days. Anyway, we managed to spruce the place up again and did all we could to make it inviting. We had a little fire put in the dining room and there was a small Victorian grate in the sitting room with a fire, and it looked like an old-fashioned show house. Just before the door bell rang, I noticed in the kitchen a tiny little vase containing some half dead flowers which I thought spoilt the immaculate view. I quickly popped them in the oven to get them out of sight. As we stood chatting and looking at the very functional kitchen there sat my vase of flowers looking at us through the oven door! Fortunately the prospective buyers wanted to buy the house straight away.

I've always had a strong mix of personality. I'm very confident, yet at times I completely lack it. I feel good about who I am and proud of my achievements, yet sometimes I feel embarrassed, inadequate and guilty. At times I feel tough and unbreakable; yet again there is another side to this where I feel frightened and vulnerable.

I've been known to put on a front that just isn't true. I suppose an example of this was when my Dad died. His funeral was held on a Tuesday afternoon, and so that morning I ran my market stall as usual, asking permission from the market superintendent to pack up and leave early. I remember washing my hands and face at my Mum's house a few minutes before we were due to leave and her bringing me her smart sheepskin coat to put on. I hadn't even thought to change. I was in such denial throughout his three month battle with stomach cancer that I continued to be cheerful and 'normal 'when visiting. I had my moments of complete despair, but mostly I would behave as if nothing was happening, even though my dad was the light of my life and my hero, and I know the feeling was the same towards all his kids. Years later my eyes would leak if I thought about him. He was 57 years old when he died. Most days I still think about my dad, and I drive Dave 'up the wall' because I repeat all his sayings. 'Let your eye be your guide', 'You reap what you sow'. If I say any of Dad's sayings Dave sighs and says "Thanks very much, Bill," even though he's never met him.

My mother never recovered from the death of my father. She tried to get involved in things like helping at the luncheon club for the elderly, bowling and socialising. My Aunt would say "Your mum and dad were like bread and butter; they went together". There was always a feeling of emptiness once my dad had departed.

We had lived in Foulsham for about a year and, having made a good profit from renovating the house, planned our next project which would be a property that would enable us to provide care in the community. One day we were driving into Kings Lynn and by chance noticed the Old Mill House at Gayton was for sale. Dave was not keen because he thought there was no land attached, but with a bit of my "gentle persuasion" we went and had a look. It was the perfect place. It had previously been used as a bed and breakfast and was currently up for sale due to bankruptcy. In fact both the old Mill House and the Mill tower itself were for sale; the Mill House for £42,000. This was way beyond our price range but my mother lent us the extra money we needed which took us seven years to pay back.

We decided to explore all avenues of care and Dave, already being a social worker, had the necessary knowledge. I was selling second hand clothes on a market stall and really liked the idea of working with people, which is something I love and seem to a have a flair for. The idea of working together with Dave was exciting and would be fun, but what could we do? We explored care of the elderly by visiting a home where my aunt worked but it didn't appeal. I think our first choice would have been children in care or leaving care, but to be honest there was so much red tape and it just looked so complicated we decided against it. We visited County Hall in Norwich and had a conversation with the Homes Registration department who showed us a map of East Anglia and the areas of need. We liked the idea of West Norfolk and luckily for us there was absolutely no mental health provision in or around the Kings Lynn area.

To be quite honest I had no idea what "mental health" meant but I didn't really care because to me people are people regardless of the label put on them. My 'gut instinct' was to provide care for people with mental health problems. I wanted the business to be an extension of my family but at the same time earn us 'a few quid'. I supposed it would be a bit like 'adult fostering'.

Once our plan was decided my determination took over. The house in Foulsham was sold and although we were hoping for a smooth transition into the Mill House with our two lads, Shane and Lee, it was not to be. Due to the previous owner's bankruptcy matters we were unable to move straight in and had to rent a property in Flitcham for about two months. Eventually it was sorted out and we arrived. The children were running about, getting lost in the building and we quickly became aware of how big it was. How were we going to afford to run it? We couldn't even afford to put the heating on, let alone fill the oil tank, but it felt very exciting!

Over the next few months we consulted with the Highways Department, Planning Department, Building Control, Environmental Health and Home's Registration. Only the latter thought it was a good idea! Highways feared the road was too busy and dangerous. Planners didn't want it because the neighbourhood had got wind of our plans. Local hysteria brewed and a petition was going round the village which led to an article on the front page of the local press. The flavour was along the lines of 'keep these mental health people locked away, we don't want to be stabbed in our beds'. What they did not realize was that once I get the bit between my teeth and am determined to achieve something, nothing puts me off. In fact the opposite, I love a challenge. Despite the whispering campaign in the village and being 'blanked' at the school gates we plodded on with our plan. We eventually had to enlist outside help and employed a retired Chief Executive of the Planning Committee. He did a fantastic job and without his intervention I would not have this story to tell. We eventually appealed to the Secretary of State for a hearing to settle all the opposition from Highways, Planning etc. The only support we received was from the Home's Registration Department who believed there was a need for community support for people with mental health problems.

In fact it took about a year before we were ready to start. Within that year we were, to say the least, in financial difficulty. I used to head off to my jumble sales and collect as many treasures as I could and then resell on Tuesday Market in Kings Lynn, Fakenham market on Thursday and Holt on a Friday. Dave continued to work as a social worker in Norwich but his wage wasn't sufficient to cover our costs. So life wasn't easy, but we had a tremendous amount of fun and what a scream we had at times! Life was hilarious!

We advertised for Bed and Breakfast which brought all sorts of characters to our door. We had a big wood fire that we couldn't afford to feed and so we used to go out 'wooding' with our trailer into nearby woods, with our two boys helping, and taking it back so we could all keep warm. The Bed and Breakfast industry was not quite as straightforward as it at first seemed. The house had been used in the past for B & B which included a package for people to come and restore furniture whilst staying in the main house. This meant it hadn't got an independent reputation for offering accommodation.

We lived in the house for one year before we finally got permission to open for residential care. The year was certainly not wasted and we had a couple of residents move in as lodgers, unbeknown to our B & B guests. We certainly had quite a challenging time one way or another with hordes of officials coming round to turn their noses up as to why we couldn't have this or that. They could not understand a community group of people with mental health problems living in a small village like Gayton. Eventually everything was passed.

In the early days a young lad moved in with us who I will call Ant. Dave used to work with young offenders on an alternative to custody scheme. Young people were sent to work on various projects in the community and had to live at a residential placement near Fakenham as an alternative to custody. We took in Ant because he had nowhere to go when the scheme finished. He had quite a lot of problems, mainly due to the fact that he was a naughty teenager as opposed to a criminal. We gave him the opportunity to do some growing up in a safe environment. I have to say he did push me to the limits! Although I was immensely fond of him I had this fantasy of how people should behave and how we could encourage people to grow and make positive changes.

Let me give you some examples of the type of behaviour we were confronted with which provided us with our first learning curve. Firstly, we had a private telephone with a little box beside it which said 'if anyone other than family used the telephone please pop some money in the box to help cover the costs of your call'. I came downstairs at 3am one morning and found Ant sitting on the stairs with the phone swinging between his legs, having used it to make random phone calls. One of these was having a little chat with people in Australia which landed us with the most astronomical phone bill. We quickly realised that we needed a phone lock. Needless to say he picked that phone lock so we had yet again another enormous phone bill. I think we got something more sophisticated after that! On another occasion he asked to paint his bedroom which I thought was a really great idea and what a nice thing to do for a young lad; give him his own space and let him express himself. He decided to paint it black with white and silver stars on the ceiling. That was not a problem, so we went out and bought various tins of paint and set him up with a stepladder and dust sheets over his bed. We offered to give him a hand but he declined as he was keen to do it himself. I warned him to be careful and to make a neat job of it but within about fifteen minutes of leaving him to it he had moved the steps with the tin of paint on top which tipped straight over onto the floor. He then walked through the paint in his socks and all the way down the stairs to tell me what had happened. There was wet white paint everywhere, but we didn't make too much of it and cleaned him up.

He was full of mischief. One night he woke us at 3am by banging on our bedroom door and running away. We then went through to the main living area to see what was going on and we were confronted by the kitchen table full of food that he'd made as a feast for us. He was sitting under the table laughing heartily. These were the kind of 'little jollies' that were a regular occurrence and in fact he was probably one of the only residents who would make steam come out of my ears! I'm sure he was sent to test my self-control because I had always had a fairly short fuse as a youngster, being a feisty individual! He used to go across to our village shop and take out umpteen videos on our rental card and sit and watch them. The shop would phone and ask him to return the films he had borrowed but he was so disrespectful; he couldn't care less whether he took the videos back or not.

On another occasion he found work for a few days and he earned some money. With his wages he bought a new push bike and set off into the village to have a drink at the local pub. We felt comfortable with him coming and going as he pleased on the understanding that he usually returned around eleven o'clock. We didn't know where he was going but we thought things were going pretty well and we were quite proud of his efforts. Unfortunately, with money in his pocket things went a bit awry, and by eleven o'clock he hadn't returned so we went to bed. At about half past one in the morning the doorbell rang. Dave went to investigate and promptly called for me. We were confronted with Ant standing at the front door accompanied by a policeman. Ant was as white as a ghost, clearly as drunk as a skunk wearing a lady's nightdress, 'bovver' boots, and no trousers. I think he had lost his trousers, or had an accident in them, and decided to help himself to something off somebody's washing line. He had got so drunk he had lost his bike and his wallet and in his drunken state couldn't actually find his way home. He thought he'd found the right house, managed to get in the front door, climbed the stairs, got into bed, realised that somebody was already in the bed and so took himself out of the bed, back to the landing and sat at the top of the stairs. The house owner who was in the sitting room heard somebody walking about upstairs and discovered Ant sitting at the top of the stairs in his nightdress and his 'bovver' boots looking confused and rather the worse for wear. After taking him downstairs the house owner locked him in the garage and called the police. The police arrived and despite his drunken condition managed to establish that he lived with us. Not the most helpful thing, just as we are about to open a new residential home for mental health residents. After he moved on from us he used to make regular visits, usually because he needed something, but eventually made his own life which has proved to be successful. Many years later he turned up at our bungalow with his wife and baby to introduce them to us and to tell us he was managing a retail unit in Peterborough, a position he had held for quite a few years.

It was not long before luck came our way in the guise of my brother Paul who was training to be a doctor at the local psychiatric unit and was working alongside a very well known local consultant. With a little bit of gentle persuasion from me, he asked if they had any patients who could benefit from being accommodated with us. We had no permission at that point to take in people with mental health problems but I wanted to see if we had the ability to work and live in close proximity with such challenges.

The Consultant agreed. There was a female patient in her early twenties at the unit who they felt would benefit from coming to us as a lodger. She had nowhere else to go and she came from a family with a variety of mental health issues. We awaited her arrival with great excitement.

She arrived with bandages on her arms and legs. At that point I had no idea why. I thought perhaps she had had an accident. She came in and she instantly fascinated me. She would smoke like a chimney, hardly moving the cigarette away from her lips which she seemed to purse into a funnel and would sit shrouded in a cloud of smoke. She was very heavily made up, in fact caked with make-up. She was a voluptuous looking woman, with hair that stood on end most of the time, but there was a gentleness about her and she really was quite a delight. I will call her Mrs A.

So Mrs. A moved in and all went well for a few days. I later discovered that the bandages were due to her habit of getting a razor blade and cutting through her wrists and her ankles periodically when life became difficult. She was suffering from schizophrenia. Schizophrenia is a chronic mental health condition that causes a range of different psychological symptoms. These include; hallucinations: hearing or seeing things that do not exist. Delusions: believing in things that are untrue. Hallucinations and delusions are often referred to as psychotic symptoms or symptoms of psychosis. (Psychosis is when somebody is unable to distinguish between reality and their imagination.)

At that point I had never heard of schizophrenia but that didn't really matter because I felt she was just a lady who had problems and troubles that were difficult for her to cope with. She hadn't lived with us very long when we had a phone call from a friend of ours called Colin Orchard, who was working on a film called Revolution that was being filmed in Kings Lynn. Big stars such as Donald Sutherland were involved. Colin knew how difficult life was for us financially and phoned to say that he had been speaking to three special effects men who were working on the film set, and needed accommodation for a while. He asked if we would be interested. We couldn't let such an opportunity pass us by and agreed. They seemed really nice chaps, full of life and energy, and we all seemed to click quite quickly. However, their first breakfast was absolutely hilarious. I'd set the breakfast table at the dining room end of the communal kitchen area. The main sitting and living area was seventy two feet long and mainly open plan. The men had just sat down and started tucking into their egg and bacon when in walked Mrs. A. She looked like nothing on earth; I mean these chaps are thinking that they are living in a normal family run bed and breakfast with Dave and me when in walks this lady. She entered in a full length black silk negligee with large protruding boobs, her hair standing on end, and she'd been to sleep with her heavy make-up on. She had her handbag over her shoulder and as always, a cigarette on the go.

The men turned towards her as she entered the room. She was oblivious to them sitting having their breakfast and she just walked through, not far from their table, and plonked herself down quite heavily in an armchair near to where they were sitting, continuing to smoke her cigarette in her normal distinctive way, looking very vacant, staring just directly in front of her, very spaced out. The mens' heads turned, their mouths full of egg and bacon and their eyes and their expressions a complete picture. I dropped behind the kitchen counter crying with laughter, tears running down my face, because it was like the beginning of a farce. After gathering myself together I made Mrs. A a cup of coffee and gave it to her and carried on as if everything was normal. They continued eating their breakfast with raised eyebrows and I just carried on as if Mrs. A was a regular guest.

During the twelve weeks that the special effects men were with us a second character arrived at the Mill who I will refer to as Mr. N. He was a young man suffering with schizophrenia and had recently been released from a secure unit. I had no idea what a secure unit was, but it didn't really matter because I presumed that if the professionals thought that anybody was well enough to come out of hospital, a secure unit or prison or anywhere else, then they must be okay to live in the community, so we welcomed Mr. N into our house.

Mr. N. was tortured by paranoia, believing that the voices of people on the television were communicating directly to him. Sometimes they made him laugh hysterically but more often they would fill him with anxiety, fear and dread. He also believed that people could read his thoughts which led him on one occasion to punch someone cycling towards him in the face. It was such incidents that led him to be taken into a secure unit.

Ironically he was an incredibly kind, gentle, and well educated young man in his early twenties. He was a gentle giant by nature but very intimidating when in a paranoid state. Any ordinary life event could spark off an outburst of anxiety and anger because his distorted thought patterns would cause him to misread a simple situation. For example, travelling on a bus he would catch someone's eye and think they could read his thoughts. He came from a loving and kind family who were devastated by his illness but who continued unconditionally to support him until his condition became unmanageable for him to live at home. To address this behaviour he was put on a heavy drug regime which resulted in him walking in a very stilted robotic sort of way and also looking 'spaced out'. He had a poor awareness of people around him and mainly lived in his own world.

The special effects men had no idea about Mrs A or Mr N's background because I never disclosed any information about them, believing that they deserved to live in as 'normal' an environment as possible. I have always strongly believed that nobody has the right to judge or discriminate against others. This has led to some stock phrases from me such as 'we are all the same human beings and will all end up in the same place eventually'; i.e. dead or, 'variety is the spice of life'. Over the years I have often reflected on myself and my own personality. How do we become who we are? Is it nature or nurture? I have a firm belief that I'm a strong mixture of both. I will expand on this later.

One evening after Dave and I had shared a bottle of wine with the special effects men they enquired about our other two guests. Clearly they were puzzled by the behaviour they had witnessed and about us being seemingly unaware of anything odd going on. We were therefore careful not to collude in any sort of discussion that suggested the other two guests were not to be seen as people in their own right. I preferred to describe their behaviour as perhaps 'a little eccentric'. I hope they left enriched by the experience of living for a few weeks with a diverse mix of characters.

The situation with the special effects men highlights the basis of my philosophy which is that people are people whoever they are, whatever their peculiarities, regardless of what label has been placed upon them, and they will always benefit from 'normalisation', whatever that really means.

Let me give you an example;

Over the years I have taken many residents to a local choir. On one occasion I took a beautiful woman in her forties who sang like an angel. I will call her B. She suffered from bipolar disorder (Bipolar disorder is a mood disorder, which means it affects the way we feel. People with bipolar disorder have elevated moods: they can be abnormally happy, but sometimes irritable. They can be over-active and full of energy, but this feeling can become so intense it becomes a problem. Most people who are bipolar suffer from both elevated and depressed moods so often it can be difficult to manage life because they never know whether they are going to be feeling high or low.)

As in any group of people an individual's emotions can vary from high to low. On one occasion the atmosphere in the hall was really buzzing because of the music. Suddenly one of the residents launched herself into a free spirited dance around the room. I was aware of some puzzled eye contact from some members of the choir but they quickly became comfortable with it because it was so emotionally uplifting. To finish the choir session at the end of an evening we used to hold hands in a circle and improvise individually which could be very emotionally charged. One evening we were improvising and B suddenly began to 'sing in tongues'. Until you have experienced this it is hard to describe the effect it can have on others! It is interesting that such behaviour can easily be seen as eccentric or odd but in fact I am aware that on many occasions emotionally high quirky behaviour could be exhibited, covertly or overtly, by me or other members of the choir! That is why I believe so strongly that everyone's experience is individual to them and should not be judged by others.

Let her tell you, in her own words, the experience one of the residents had at a choir Christmas party:

"The thoughts that would go through my head would often lead to behaviour that other people found a little odd. There was however some measure of logic if you dug deep enough.

A typical example was the Big Heart and Soul Christmas party. Social events were occasions when I often felt stressed, so when things got under way I slipped out to calm myself with some solitude and night air. Feeling at the time that my social inadequacy warranted punishment I suddenly was gripped with a compelling urge to emulate the example of self flagellation set by Sir Lancelot. Through the process of beating myself I would, so I was convinced, purify myself of my failings. I looked around for a suitable stick in the undergrowth outside but found nothing. Instead, not being deterred, I leant down in my cerise velvet dress and rolled vigorously in a rough patch of nettles. Feeling suitably chastised and smarting somewhat I returned to the village hall blissfully unaware that half of Castle Acres undergrowth was stuck to the fabric of my dress, sprouting out of my hair and trailing around my ankles. Helen took one look at me and collapsed into a fit of giggles.

"Am I mad?" I asked Helen some time later. "No" she replied, "just a little bizarre"."

CHAPTER TWO

Mr. N sparked off my curiosity about what mental illness is really about.
I think in retrospect that was when I began to leave my naivety behind and started to get my teeth into how I could be more effective.

It was clear that I couldn't keep watching Mr. N wondering if he was going to react badly to the television or the radio because that caused a lot of other problems that affected the residents. So I went about finding out about schizophrenia. I obtained lots of information from various sources, to educate myself as much as anything else, because I had no idea what it was about not having any mental health background whatsoever. Mr N clearly didn't know anything about it; in fact he didn't realize that he was schizophrenic. So although he had been through the hospital system I don't think anyone had actually told him there was a name attached to his illness. He could, by gaining information, be reassured and have a better understanding of what was happening to him. At that time Mental Health Professionals appeared to have deemed this not important, therefore denying him an opportunity to understand himself. I am not convinced as to how much this has improved. Mr N needed to be reassured that his odd behaviour was a symptom of an illness and should be seen in that context, not that he was simply 'mad' which he would often ask me if he was!

To emphasise how important the involvement of the patient can be let me share a letter with you sent by one of my ex residents to the local health authority. These are her words;

'I am writing to express my concerns at the current procedure of 'Professionals' Meetings' and in particular the meeting about myself which took place on Friday 30th August 2003.
As a service user, currently being subject to this procedure, I thought it may be useful to you, perhaps for future reference to understand a service user's view on these meetings.

Firstly, may I point out that perhaps by inviting the client you are discussing, your questions, concerns or queries may be more easily clarified and resolved. I have the capacity to understand such issues and feel that I could provide the most relevant information, having been acquainted with my thought processes and behaviour for the past 28 years. Understandably, I do comprehend that in the past I may have been unable to make lucid decisions but this is a rarity and not the 'normal' or current situation. Society already isolates and excludes people suffering from mental health problems and I feel that professionals working within this field should be aware that possibly these meetings are displaying the same sort of effect.

I believe in the philosophy of empowerment and cannot understand how such practice is empowering people to make their own decisions and express their own opinions or viewpoints. I also believe that my opinions and choices are just as valid if not more so when broaching the subject of my care and my future. I do not have any kind of disability which affects my intelligence; therefore I am quite competent at being a part of any decision making. You may very well be the 'professionals' but I am the 'expert' when it comes to my own life and choices and I would therefore be very grateful to be included in such and it's my conviction that allowing this would also be extremely beneficial to the eventuality of independent living in the community.

I am aware that you may consider 'Professionals' Meetings' important in order to offer me the best care, and I do appreciate this, but equality in society, relationships and decision making, I think, are the best place to start.

I do hope that you understand my point of view and I thank you for your time.

Yours sincerely

c.c ... Consultant Psychiatrist

......CPN, MHCST
......Manager (residential Unit)'

I began to see that my need to 'normalise' and not 'label' people needed to be rethought.

I began to see that sometimes it can be useful. Try imagining what it would be like being diabetic and not knowing or being able to find anything out about it.

To return to the matter of Mr. N, it needs to be said that he was highly intelligent and academically successful at grammar school. He could be very engaging and amusing when he wasn't troubled by his voices and distorted thought patterns. So between us we started learning about schizophrenia. We looked at other peoples' histories and stories, things that had happened to them, and he seemed to gain considerable reassurance from this. One of his passions was watching football on the television. However, he became fixated by the television and began to believe people on it were talking to him. He started to believe that he was responsible for world disasters and other tragedies. As part of the education around his illness I encouraged him to take responsibly for dealing with his agitation and suggested he got up and turned the TV off himself. He did try to do this but a number of times I found him within a foot of the television screen peering in at the images to be sure they weren't talking to him before he switched it off. Can you imagine how overwhelming this can be when you truly believe something is real?

Unfortunately, this strategy impinged on other residents who were watching the television and was not fair to them once he became agitated. Clearly this strategy was only partially successful.

So we devised plan B which consisted of increasing his self awareness and finding ways of diverting him into positive activities.

I suggested that he thought about what was happening to him, that it was part of his illness and people on the telly were not talking to him. Sometimes that was really difficult for him, because his beliefs were so solid. At other times with a bit of help we could bring him back to some kind of reality. I remember one Sunday afternoon he was watching football and getting extremely agitated from perceived messages coming from the pitch. He didn't like physical exercise but on this particular day I put my hand on his shoulder and told him we were going for a walk. I had my stern teacher face on that said there was no negotiating; we were going for a walk. Much to his disgruntlement we went for a 'route march' of a walk. A common trait I soon discovered with people suffering from troubled and distorted thought patterns was a tendency to miss the world around them because of their mental preoccupations. As a result he would walk with his head down looking at the ground. To counteract this I encouraged him to look at the beauty around us. I just felt that this was a much healthier course of action than being upset. He used to be very unmotivated and lethargic, and I hope I didn't bully him but I certainly wouldn't take no for an answer. Gradually, I got him involved in a variety of activities. I taught him to cook, albeit a very simple diet. We used to go to Sainsbury's and I would support him in choosing what he needed for the week.

Each week we would write a menu together. His choices were limited because he was very fussy. In the store we would collect a basket of food which he seemed to enjoy. He started to establish simple routines that he managed well. This included attendance at a day centre in Kings Lynn two or three times a week. He would cook for himself each day; he was into the local football team and would go and watch Kings Lynn football team play, home and away. He also enjoyed our village football team games and would regularly kick a ball in the field with our boys. Our aim was to provide a focus and purpose that gave him reason to get up every day. I think by giving him blunt consistent messages he was reminded that he had a responsibility for himself and others. I think this gave him reassurance and put his feet firmer on the ground. This was enhanced by an incredible amount of support and work from Dave. When Mr N first moved in with us, he dreamed of having his own flat, and if you'd met him you would have thought that this was unlikely given his mental state. However, two years later he had improved sufficiently to achieve his dream. Every year without fail he sends me a Christmas card. Periodically he calls in to see us to say hello and, bearing in mind it was well over twenty years ago, it is quite remarkable that he has kept up the contact. One day I bumped into him in Sainsbury's and I couldn't believe my eyes. I noticed that his selection of groceries were the same as they had been all those years before. I was surprised that he was still buying the same crisps, ice cream, burgers, chips, and fruit; in fact everything in the basket was as we used to buy, and that was twenty years ago. He has done amazingly well and has never returned to hospital since leaving the Mill which is remarkable and all credit to him.

In the early days before our registration Mr. N and Mrs A were lodgers and were paying the minimum to stay with us which did not cover the cost of providing their care. Dave continued to work in Norwich and every Thursday I continued to sell second hand clothes on Fakenham market. Mr. N and Mrs. A had to be cared for twenty four hours a day which meant they used to have to come with me. We would see it as a 'jolly'. Mr. N would usually go to the Day Centre but occasionally would come with me and quickly become bored and sometimes agitated. Luckily, the Fakenham Market was only a half day. They would both sit behind me in deckchairs. Mrs A would drink copious amounts of tea with a 'fag' constantly on the go. Mr. N would wander about drinking coke, eating burgers and not really helping. I did try to encourage them to take part but they lacked the ability to concentrate.

Mrs. A. had experienced a very difficult life; she'd come from a large family and there were hereditary factors of schizophrenia within her family group. She and her siblings experienced deprivation in lots of ways, they had little money and their parents' complex personalities led to inadequate parenting which at times was unwittingly cruel. In the first twelve months that Mrs. A lived with us, she made twelve suicide attempts which were very distressing for everybody but what a tremendous learning curve for me. At that time my understanding of mental health was still in the early stages and I relied on my instinctive reactions. When I was growing up my father used to say "Helen use your mother nature instincts and let your eye be your guide".

This has stood me in good stead. Mrs A taught me a phenomenal amount about observational skills, body language, and the value of noting what wasn't being said rather than what was being said. I would always encourage her to speak openly of the troubles and distresses that she had as a result of her schizophrenia. Her medication was a slow release drug by injection fortnightly administered by a Community Psychiatric Nurse. This reduced some of the extreme behaviour but created unwelcome side effects such as joint stiffness, involuntary body movements and insatiable thirst. Her behaviour was dependent upon her thought processes which varied according to the stress factors at the time which could be the voices in her head working for or against her. She could therefore experience negative and destructive feelings, but being a very passive and gentle individual, would internalise this and not express it openly in a healthy manner. Consequently she would, at times, cut herself severely.

Her thoughts and ideas were inevitably extreme. What she wanted from her life was at times unrealistic and changeable. Once, she packed her bags preparing to go to London to become a prostitute. A few days later she would be packed ready to go again but this time to be a nun. Her illness prevented her from developing proper self awareness, thereby leaving her constantly confused. She could at times be a bizarre character. She was a fanatical smoker but her budget was not sufficient to support her habit. Therefore she never had enough cigarettes. One night she went across to the Crown, our local pub. She had put on her smart clothes, had her hair done, and applied her heavy make-up. She entered the pub and proceeded to walk round from table to table emptying the ashtrays into her handbag so that she could return home and make some roll ups. In fact, before she'd even left the pub, she had sat on a rug in front of a beautiful open fire and started splitting the dog ends up until the landlady suggested that she left, having informed us of the situation. This may have been her version of recycling but she returned to the Mill totally unfazed as usual.

Over the years Dave and I were very grateful for the kindness and understanding we received from the Managers of The Crown who displayed so much tolerance towards our residents. The Crown was a very middle class pub with hunting/shooting/fishing clientele but their approach towards our residents has always been appreciated.

One night we were all seated eating at the dinner table when Mrs A left the table and went to sit at the far end of the open plan sitting room. I just happened to hear a noise from that direction and when I investigated I discovered she had put a plastic bag over her head that was then being very tightly sucked onto her face as she breathed. I went over to her and pushed my fingers through the bag where her mouth and nose was, ripped the bag, pulled it off her head and I said "Look, you're out of order, you don't really need to do that kind of stuff here, you know we've got family, we've got kids, it's just not appropriate, stop it!" I attempted to increase her self awareness but the destructive behaviour continued. However, despite her behaviour she was a lovely and harmless soul.

A major turning point was when she decided she wanted a hamster. We thought this was a great idea but took time to explain that she would have to think about her behaviour more because she would be responsible for a living creature. Marmalade duly arrived. It became her pride and joy and was like her child.

Her horrible experiences continued and I remember one day she was on a bus going to visit her parents. Whilst on the bus she was hallucinating, seeing dead bodies in the dykes along the road. She got off the bus at her destination and immediately rang me from a phone box to tell me about it because she was so frightened. I was so pleased to receive that call because it demonstrated that she had been able to talk to me about it and not self harm.

We talked it over and I gave her some very firm reassurance and although I never actually said 'there, there' I did explain that it was part of her illness, that there were no bodies out there. They were not real; there was nothing out there going to hurt her and it was her illness. So to receive that call was rewarding because it indicated a level of trust and faith in us.

Mrs. A considered the hamster as her baby. She cleaned her cage meticulously, she cleaned the water bottle, and she bought her presents with her weekly money. She became her family. On the days that she felt unsure of herself, I would remind her of her responsibility to Marmalade which gave her a different focus, reminding her that she had to be responsible. Mrs. A, with the hamster, finally moved on from the Mill House into a small, safe, warden controlled flat designed predominately for the elderly. This provided a gentle non threatening environment that suited her needs. I think she had developed a number of skills and learnt a lot about herself. I visited her regularly in the early days and nearly banged the door down on one occasion, shouting through the letterbox before she would open up. Sometimes she was scared, having believed she had heard voices or noises, and so would be hiding terrified under her duvet, too frightened to come out. Twenty years afterwards she was still managing to maintain an independent life style.

I recall one incident with Mrs. A which could be seen as amusing, although it was actually very sad. We had always discussed what she would do when Marmalade died and gently reminded her that animals, like people, don't last forever. On the first night of her moving into the flat she rang me and said "Helen, what am I going to do if Marmalade dies?" We had assured her that if the hamster died whilst we were at the Mill we would have a burial in the garden. Two weeks later she rang me in a very distressed state informing me Marmalade had died and so we did just that. She said she would put Marmalade in a little box and come over on the bus. The bus journey turned out to be quite eventful. Her handbags were always full of bits and pieces and she'd wrapped Marmalade up in toilet tissue and popped her on top of the bag, which she'd put on the floor of the bus.

Just before she got off the bus Marmalade had rolled off the bag and under the seat along with the myriad contents of her bag.

Her refusal to get off the bus whilst rummaging under the seat for a dead hamster did not overly impress the bus driver or the passengers.   Mrs A was unable to do anything in a hurry, possibly due to the medication she was taking. I have observed over the years that most sufferers of schizophrenia lack any awareness of the effects of their behaviour on other people. As a consequence her fellow passengers had to sit patiently whilst she rummaged, oblivious of the fact that she was delaying their journey. At the Mill we buried Marmalade, made a cross, put flowers on the grave and mourned the loss with copious cups of tea and fags. A trait of her illness seemed to be the excessive amounts of tea and cigarettes she could consume in a short space of time.

We discussed her getting another hamster which she could call Marmalade 2nd as she had proved that she could provide safety, security, love and affection for an animal.   This would also continue to give her a focus and something to look forward to, something I believe we all need. Shortly after, we went to the pet shop and purchased Marmalade 2nd. I haven't been in touch with her for many years now, but I occasionally see her brother and enquire about her. She maybe on Marmalade 22nd by now, who knows! I want to acknowledge the ongoing struggle people like Mrs A have every day yet manage to survive the emotional pain and discomfort that comes with their illness.

CHAPTER THREE

Sadly even under the closest scrutiny from friends, family, partners and professionals, the level of trauma and distress is sometimes undetected and becomes too much to bear and can lead to tragedy.

I want to share Matt's story with you, written by his partner and best friend, Janet. I feel Matt's story highlights the depth of this pain and its effects on those close to them.

Here is Matt's story in Janet's words;

I have written this to make sense of Matt's life which ended in suicide as a result of schizophrenia. A taboo subject that most people don't like to talk of, or can't understand. Suicide goes against our survival instinct, it occurs in an abnormal state of mind. A suicidal person has extremely restricted cognitive thinking, whereby the only option that appears to be available to end emotional or physical pain is to end life.

I first met Matt at Portland Street, a sister home of the Mill; I was a support worker and I would describe him as the 'unofficial lifter of spirits'. At first I wasn't aware that Matt had been diagnosed with schizophrenia (it's not something that is visible!!). Matt used to visit a lot and just chat happily to the residents and staff who lived there. Matt always had time for everyone. He was one of those people who has a presence - lifts a room and spreads happiness. It was hard to believe that he had had such unhappiness and pain in his own life.

Matt would also help out anybody and everybody, he had so much to give to others, and what a sense of humour.

After a while I kept hoping that Matt would pop in. I found myself really looking forward to the possibility of him turning up. I also began to see that there was much more - I began to see his intelligence, depth and uniqueness and his infectious laugh. Matt then began to spend a bit more time with me. On one particular day I was painting the back wall of the garden at the unit and Matt came out and spent the rest of the day painting it with me. I learnt a lot more about him that day. As the weeks went by I got to know him better and then Matt wasn't there any more. I was told that he was in hospital.

I found myself missing him, thinking about him all the time, missing our conversations about all aspects of life. It was then that I realized that I had fallen in love with him. I plucked up the courage to visit him in hospital, but it wasn't the same person I saw there. I saw his pain and suffering. I also saw him very medicated, and the energetic, bouncy person with the great sense of humour looked so desperately unhappy and sedated. It hurt me to see him that way.
Matt later told me that he remembered little of those weeks. A couple of weeks later Matt came to Portland Street to visit everyone. As he was leaving he said that he had missed me. And that was when I knew I meant something to him too.

On May 8th 2001 I was helping Matt move some of his things from one flat to another. We got the last load into the lift and I will never forget how he held me and kissed me for the first time and from that moment on I could not have walked away.

Matt gave me something that I never thought I would find - someone who loved me with equal intensity. If something was broken Matt fixed it. Matt fixed me. He took away the loneliness that I had felt since a fairly young age. I had met the person who was on the same emotional, intellectual and sexual wavelength. From that day on we were a bit pathetic really!! - not bearing to be apart and talking all night. It got to the point in our relationship where I could be thinking about something abstract, and Matt would know (that used to freak me out a bit!!). We didn't have to speak to just know. I was suddenly the luckiest person in the world - Matt brought so much love and laughter into our lives.

Every second of every day was precious time and we didn't want to waste any of it. Some of the most precious times were first thing in the morning, before the rush of the day began, where

Matt and I would sit on the sofa in the conservatory looking out at the garden, not really saying too much, drinking a cup of tea and feeling completely and utterly content with each other and at peace with life.

It wasn't only me that experienced the kind of love that Matt had an ability to give. My two children also experienced this love. I remember Sam's first day at his new school - Matt fussing around him, making sure everything was perfect and then seeing him get anxious waiting for Sam to come out of school to see that his first day had gone OK. Matt was very protective and loving to Dan and Sam - so much more than any father had or could be to my boys.

Matt always kept himself busy - doing things for others mostly. He worked at a day centre for adults with learning disabilities on a Friday - he was known as their Friday boy. Matt loved doing things in the house and garden and also at Portland Street. Whatever needed doing he did it. Matt was extremely nurturing - I had never felt so cared for. He had a huge ability to love others.

When Matt wasn't running around after everybody he would draw or write poems. My house is full of his art work, the things he made, the garden full of the plants and flowers that he had planted there. He also enjoyed Martial Arts.

In all these things it became clear that Matt was a perfectionist, and never really felt that anything was 'good enough', a hard judge on himself. He was a strong character, who wouldn't want others to see his vulnerabilities. These things he didn't share with me - I am aware of his past and the things that occurred but due to my loyalty to Matt and confidentiality I will keep that private.

Matt once said to me – 'Janet, no one before, no one during and no one after, only you' It later transpired that he meant it.

Matt talked about his Schizophrenia. He had been hospitalized nine times in the preceding five years. Matt had always said that he wouldn't want myself or the boys to see him if he became unwell. I told him that it would be OK - that we'd get through it - but we also both thought (wrongly) that he might just be OK. He said that he wouldn't want me to see him any differently than the Matt I knew. I told him that I would be OK too and that nothing could change the love I had for him. Matt becoming ill was just something we didn't think about - life was just too happy.

Matt didn't like to take his medication for schizophrenia - it slowed him down, sedated him and had an adverse effect on his ability to be intimate, so he didn't take it. I can't blame him really; Matt was an extremely active person who enjoyed life to the full, why would a 28 year old want those side effects? And yes they might have saved his life - might have kept him alive - but alive living half a life? No not Matt - he loved to live life to the full.

When Matt had said that he would never want myself or the boys to see him unwell I thought that he meant that he would take himself away from the area and admit himself to another hospital or not allow me to see him in hospital. Looking back I now know what he meant. Matt was not going to go through it again.

A huge risk factor for suicide is actually when life has been going well for someone and then they begin to become unwell. Life is good and they see the black abyss looming and just don't want to go down into it. I was later told that when Matt became ill he went into some very dark places. Places that Matt didn't talk to me about - he used to say that he would never want to put that on me.

We spent two very happy carefree years. It might be that a couple are together for fifty years and don't experience that kind of love. Matt was then and is now my soul mate.

A couple of weeks before he died, Matt wasn't sleeping well. He was becoming withdrawn - the war in Iraq was bothering him, he would talk about the shit things that people do to each other.

I didn't see it.

Forget Me Not

Friday 16th May 2003 - Matt and I are watching a film - he stops the film and says 'Janet, I need you to know that I love you and Dan and Sam'. We carry on watching the film.

I didn't see it.

Saturday 17th May - Matt wants to be close to me again, telling me how much he loves me - but he's very quiet for the rest of the day.

I didn't see it.

Sunday 18th May - Matt has a Tae Kwon Do competition. We come home. He says he is tired and needs to sleep. I want him to talk to me - what's wrong? He says he feels physically unwell, that things are getting on top of him and that he needs to rest. He then says he's going. Going where I ask - just going. I said - you're leaving me? Matt says no - but that he's going. I don't understand - I say 'You said you'd never leave me'. Matt says he's not leaving me - he's going.

I still didn't see it.

I cry, Matt cries. I put my arms around him and he cries more. He goes upstairs and tells the children to look after me.

He goes.

I still didn't see it.

I get in my car and try to get him to come home - the rest of the conversation will always remain private - they were the last words spoken. Matt carries on walking and I go home – devastated, still thinking that the one person who wasn't supposed to leave has left me - broken all his promises of love - I think about my own grief and loss.

I still didn't see it.

I post letters to him over the next few days telling him that I respect him wanting his space - that I love him and will always be there for him. I ring all the hospitals and bed and breakfasts thinking he's gone to rest somewhere.
I'm hurting badly.

Thursday 22nd May - I go to his flat - I lift the letter box and smell a smell I will never forget. I have to get in - in a panic I ring people - they go in.

Matt had taken a massive overdose and had died some days before.

My whole world fell apart - I feel fear like I have never known, shocked - no, not Matt, no, no, no repeating around in my head. In and out of shock.
Emotional and physical pain, feeling like it's going to kill me.
Day and night meaning nothing; screaming for him, wanting to die to be with him. No, I can't be without you, I can't.
Why? Why? Why? Guilt - I didn't see. Anger, emptiness, lonely again.
The luckiest person to nothing - as quickly as that.
No one being able to take the pain away - who else can I blame?
People trying to help.
Coward or courageous?
'But he left you to find him dead, Janet' - but he didn't mean to - he didn't think that far ahead. It would have only been me though.
The note - the note I know he wrote - he would.
Dan's face crumbling, tears when I told him, Sam not letting anyone near him, Sam out of control. Matt the person who was stability, became unstable and left - he promised he wouldn't.
Words that hurt; 'We're doing the post mortem now'.
You can't see him - too disturbing - I just want to hold his hand. 'No, we won't let you'
People asking why - how do I know?
The funeral out of my hands - talking about Matt's schizophrenia at the funeral, not about Matt, but about how it was his fault because he hadn't taken his medication.

Matt who was so full of life - in a coffin. He shouldn't be there.

I now have to live the rest of my life - knowing that I didn't see it, missing him and not being able to talk to him.

Matt used to like to write poems and stories. I always told him that his poems were really good but he lacked confidence in himself. After his death some of the poems were published - I wish he'd been able to share that. It was one of the things I wanted to do for him, for him to be remembered as the talented person he was. It's also why I knew that in those last hours of despair he would have written to me - he would want me to understand. Instead I was tortured over the 'whys' that come with suicide. The 'if I could have stopped him, or seen what was coming', that comes with suicide.

I knew he would have written me a note when he died. I kept asking the coroner but he said there was only a book of poems. This was returned to his family after his death. Seven weeks after his death it was posted to me. Turning the book upside down and reading from the back pages was his suicide note telling me why. And telling myself, Dan and Sam that he loved us. Words I had so desperately needed to hear in those seven weeks. Maybe I wouldn't have felt the overwhelming desire to kill myself and to have that last conversation with Matt.

In that suicide note Matt had an opportunity to express his last words to me - I have never had that chance - but I have always known what I would say - if I had known it was his last day on Earth. Maybe I would even have understood and accepted that he could no longer live with the mental torture that is schizophrenia. No matter how much we think we understand, we can't possibly understand what it is like to live with the emotional pain and torture that schizophrenia can bring. If a cancer sufferer had fought cancer countless times over and it came back again - who are we to say that the person must endure it again? We have a right to end our emotional and physical suffering. But people also have the right to be helped as much as possible to explore other options first. I know I would have done everything to stop him - he knew that too – that's why he couldn't say 'Janet, I'm going to kill myself'.

Whilst the experience I had with Matt was the happiest time in my life and the most intense, his death was the most intense pain that I had ever felt. It was the kind of grief that feels like it will kill you. More painful than that, was telling my boys and seeing their world falling apart. Occasionally I have felt angry at Matt for the pain caused to my boys, but I know that I'm actually angry at a horrible illness called schizophrenia that kills one in ten of its victims by suicide.

In writing this I have felt that same pain - it's something I try to avoid because it is terrifying. I have to be strong; I am strong for my boys without whom I wouldn't be here today. To those people who kept me going and to one who saved my life and you know who you are - thank you from the bottom of my heart. Matt would be angry at me if I hadn't carried on.

Matt said in his suicide note that he would watch out for me if he goes to a place that allows that.

I feel that he does, that he's with me and my boys. My two boys that I am so proud of - that despite their pain have become two of the nicest people I know. Matt would be proud too. We were blessed to have him in our lives.

Five years on, there has been some healing - I have also had happiness and sadness. I know that Matt would want me to be happy - he was a beautiful person who was upset by others' suffering. I will always want that last conversation, just to say;

Matt, I love you. I am so sorry that I didn't see - didn't stop it - didn't see how you were suffering. I sit in the conservatory, I close my eyes and I imagine you're sitting quietly next to me. I feel you around me - whatever comes and goes - you will always be my soul mate. Do you remember, you imagined me and you sitting on a cloud holding hands? One day we will and I'll lie next to you once again and you'll stroke my hair until I fall asleep, pain won't exist any more and we'll just feel the love and happiness. I'll die when I'm an old woman with grey hair and when/if there is something else - I'll be heading towards you. I remember one particular time - you held me in your arms and I could have died there and then knowing that I had felt that kind of love, that hug will last until I can hold you again - yours forever, Janet.

Depending on the severity of the illness we can illustrate that the more fortunate can survive this illness. Let me describe what happened to Lorna, a thirty two year old woman, who in 2000 moved into one of the sister houses to the Mill who has managed to maintain independence. Lorna suffered from schizophrenia and felt terrified and isolated by her hallucinations, thought disorders, and fear. There was a lack of clarity for her as to what was wrong with her. It was not until she came to us that she received a proper diagnosis of schizophrenia and treatment appropriate to her needs. The treatment was holistic and included a professional health support team, Psychiatrist, CPN, staff and key workers from the home. Lorna also found other residents who had similar experiences to her reassuring. She found safety in her new home environment which she described as 'living as part of the Waltons'. She told me she felt an unspoken bond with staff and residents which she described as 'a close knit sisterhood' and camaraderie where she regained her confidence. Lorna has since confided to me that without this intervention she would probably be dead. Her relationships with her family improved once she became less dependent on them. So often the unwell child or person will have unrealistic expectations of family and friends or people who are close to them.

It has been my experience that parents suffer their child's pain, know tremendous guilt and feel powerless around their child's mental anguish. Being a parent myself of four boys and experiencing the normal stresses of them growing up, I fully empathise with parents who have to cope with the more extreme behaviour resulting from mental illness. I take my hat off to them.

Undoubtedly mental illness is traumatic and sometimes tragic but it can nevertheless have its lighter, more humorous moments. Here is a snapshot from Lorna;

Dealing with paranoid schizophrenia has never been an easy ride. There have been some really scary moments but equally some funny ones too.

During one episode of psychosis I went for a five hour walk along the beach. As I was walking my delusional thinking took hold. I believed I was Jesus (OK I know I'm female!). While I was walking I thought I was saving the world, saving Africa from poverty, establishing world peace and all the other issues that burden this planet. I came across a little stream. I stopped and pondered. A little voice was telling me "Hey, you are Jesus, you can walk on water", and as the water seeped through my shoes and clothes the little voice in my head said "it must be your day off."

On another occasion I believed there was a conspiracy theory going on. At this point I was living in a hostel. The theory was that I was bugged and the hostel was too. I went to the Manager, who thought it was hilarious. At this point I didn't know I was talking in whispers. By this time the Manager was getting worried and called over a very posh, immaculate woman who was quite elderly and happened to be on the board of directors. Again I was talking in whispers and when this lady arrived she asked me what was wrong. You must remember that I was sure this woman was bugged and that MI5 wanted me. This elderly lady had just come from the hairdressers. I was convinced she had a bugging device in her hair and without thinking twice I began rifling through her hair. I then realised there was no bugging device to be found but after I had finished her hair looked like a bird's nest! The sweet thing was that she took it in her stride and was really nice to me. I laugh so much when I think back to that.

During another one of my episodes I was in a psychiatric ward. I thought I was having telepathic conversations with Bill Clinton. I was convinced it was real. I don't know anything about politics but every so often I would talk to the same nurse about what Bill had to say to me. I remember one telepathic message and that was the world was coming to an end and Bill had said that I just had to 'say the word' and it would end. Well I told the nurse that in five minutes the world would end and when it didn't happen I went to her again and said 'in the next five minutes' and nothing happened. I must have kept this up all night and to this day I don't know how that nurse kept a straight face!

Lorna has elegantly described how her illness affected her. I would add that the extreme medication used to treat schizophrenia can be highly successful but carries the risk that the sufferer, once feeling free of the symptoms, ceases to take their medication and the symptoms then return. This can lead to the individual being admitted to hospital for their own safety and the medication restarted. One of the cornerstones of our philosophy at the Mill was to allow individuals the freedom of choice. This included accepting there were occasions when we would support someone stopping their medication as a free choice. This was a risky decision and we did not take it lightly, having first carefully assessed any major risk to the individual's well being. This was underpinned by a safety package drawn up between us and the individual which consisted of a quick intervention by staff if unwarranted signs and symptoms began to reoccur.

Having said that there are individuals who can be of danger to themselves, and rarely others, and with whom we had a constant battle to help them overcome their lack of insight and awareness of the need to take their medication in order to have any quality in their life.

Sadly, for some even with or without medication their quality of life was limited and 'wellness' unsustainable.

I need to address the involvement of parents in a little more depth as I believe it is so important in building a picture of how mental illness affects everyone involved with the individual.

At times I have experienced enormous frustration at a parent's unwitting sabotage of their child's journey back to health of which medication has played a vital part. Very often parents expected an unrealistically swift recovery, which was invariably not the case. However, at times it would be weeks, months or years to achieve a recovery. It was sad at times to witness a parent waiting and hoping for their child to be returned to them 'as they used to be' before the illness.

I can only imagine what life must feel like when one of your children is struck by mental illness; a bout of mental stress is bad enough. Failure at getting the university place they were hoping for, not getting the job they wanted, ending of a loving relationship, bereavement and so on. There are many reasons why our 'mood' gets down and we struggle to 'pull ourselves together' – always a favourite catch phrase! But what about people who get stuck, the doom and despair never letting up? Or the confusion of not knowing what reality is. Have you ever been really frightened? Imagine if it never went away or was always coming back and you never knew when. This is what happens to some people who endure mental illness. They can't stop the roundabout and get off, it just won't stop. In my experience it's difficult enough for the individual to cope with their mental health problems, but so often parents are tortured too. They blame themselves; they question where they went wrong. They ask themselves what could have been done differently. Mental illness does not discriminate against who it captures. Many people I have worked with over the years have been abandoned by friends and family. The needs of some ill people are relentless, unreasonable and not achievable. The support system around them eventually gets worn down, fragments and disintegrates.

Parents have displayed so many mixed emotions. They desperately try to rescue their distressed child rather than giving them straight, honest messages. They collude with distorted thought patterns and disruptive ideas in the hope they might make their deluded child feel better. They give unnecessary financial support rather than allowing their child to manage and take responsibility for their own finances. They offer money, and material things are given because a parent feels guilty or helpless. They give mixed messages; they say no, no, no to something and then say yes. Boundaries that need to be clear become 'woolly' and detrimental. Washing, ironing and cleaning remain the responsibility of the parents. In their eyes it would be the least they could do under the circumstances. One family made constant promises to their child that they would more often than not break. Parents would condemn the much needed medication that their child was prescribed, thinking that it made them worse. One father told his slowly recovering daughter "I'm never in favour of filling anyone with unnecessary medication", but for most people it was a necessity to have some semblance of a 'normal' life. Parents sometimes encourage their child to stop taking medication. What some refused to realize was that getting well takes time and there are no magic wands for instant cures. Life is not something that happens to us, it belongs to each individual. Our treatment and responses need to be tailor made, unique, creative and under constant assessment. How are parents, guardians or supporters expected to manage this? It's a 'tall order'. It may be needed for years. I'm not sure how much support is out there for parents. I plan to look into it in my retirement. I can't imagine how I would feel or react if one of my children became the 'chosen one' because that's exactly how it is. Don't ever think it happens to others and won't happen to you. We don't know how we would react if in this situation. I have seen the most unlikely of families fall apart under the pressure. I can't start to tell you how sad it has made me feel watching loving families fall apart under the strain. Often by the time a young adult came into our care, the damage was done. Carers had been pushed to the limit. Expectations had sometimes been put onto them from professional services because of lack of resources. They had to wait too long for help and support. Their own determination has tried to see the problem through. The carer has 'burnt themselves out'; they have no energy left and find themselves feeling fragile. However, sometimes dealing with health difficulties means that families pull together and become united.

I have always tried to include parents and carers in decision making if the resident feels it appropriate. This way I could be very straight in my approach and encourage all concerned to pursue the same path and strive towards rehabilitation in an agreed strategy.

Sometimes I would feel disappointed and let down. One such occasion was when we accommodated a young girl, whose parents were financially comfortable, having worked very hard building their own company. They would have regular contact with staff and their daughter. When she arrived at the Mill it was like having a whirlwind arrive. She was stunningly attractive inside and out. She could 'charm the birds out of the trees', especially if she wanted her own way. She had lived in the city and had been a 'party animal'. Late nights, long weekends, drinking and smoking cannabis had led her to feel thought disordered and out of control. Her loving parents, family and friends would encourage her to visit and stay over with them most weekends. I soon said that a visit once in a while would be more beneficial as on her return she would be back to square one. She would leave on a Friday or Saturday and return on a Sunday having had lots of unhealthy stimulation leaving her unwell and out of control. Once I invited her mum and sister in when they returned her on a Sunday evening. Our resident was looking pale and tired. We discussed together the weekend she had had. "We had a laugh" they all agreed. It turned out they had gone clubbing the Saturday night having shared a few 'joints' before hitting the night club where they downed a few vodkas – this included her mum! I never want to be judge and jury. I don't wear a halo myself and I loved a good smoke in my youth. But this young woman had already had mental health problems leading to trouble with the police and paranoia and anxiety. And in front of me I had her mum telling me that they were just having a 'laugh'. I told them very clearly, in my opinion, what they needed to do to aid a full recovery before it was too late. My advice was systematically ignored. I felt for her mum; she wanted to support her daughter on one level but didn't have the capacity not to over indulge her and stick to decisions and boundaries. She colluded with her daughter's bad behaviour and made excuses for her. In the end I gave her notice to leave. Not because she was an unpleasant girl, not because she had an unpleasant family but because the lack of boundaries and destructive interactions made it impossible to work with this family and their daughter. I could see the situation was on a downhill spiral and I was not prepared to be on board – six weeks after leaving she was back on the ward.

To complete this chapter I will end with an account of a very dear friend of mine whose experience illustrates the pain that parents can go through.

To put into context the arbitrary nature of mental illness I must explain that this family were high achievers, one of whom was highly successful in the music business, and one of her children went on to gain a first at University. Her two children she refers to were twins, both of whom appeared well until they completed their exams at sixteen. It is recognised that the onset of schizophrenia occurs between fifteen and thirty five and can be triggered by stress. Both boys developed this illness within months of each other. This incident increases the likelihood that this illness is not only hereditary but an organic defect within the brain. Both boys were physically fit, talented sportsmen, but not now sadly.

Rose's story:
The first time I heard of the Mill was in unusual circumstances, although I had passed it many times driving to Kings Lynn, rising like a light house from the rural village of Gayton. At the time I ran a bookstall for my then husband on the Tuesday Market Place. Next to me was a lively bubbly girl with a wicked sense of humour selling second hand clothes. Her name was Helen. We were market traders who clicked. On a typical Tuesday market morning, Helen first mentioned the Mill. They were having great difficulty in getting it up and running due to opposition from the local community. I sympathised, and little did I know at that time how significant it would become to us. Their determination and belief brought results and they won the battle. An amazing victory. It became the main provider for respite and after care for the vulnerable.

In its infancy I worked some hours there and the atmosphere was relaxed and therapeutic. Gradually the Mill expanded and sister houses opened, all of which had the same philosophy of care and nurture.

Many years later, I met Helen in Swaffham unexpectedly outside a jumble sale. My world had been shattered and was never to be the same again. One of my twin sons was very ill with a breakdown and in the Fermoy Unit, the local psychiatric unit. His behaviour was strange and bizarre. My desperation and anxiety were apparent and typically Helen offered any help and support she could give. A life line I knew I could hang onto.

Months of confusion followed. My son, barely 17, had his whole life torn apart. Later he said "his head had exploded". We all felt we were in a harrowing play, not knowing which lines came next. I knew there was no time for tears, although my womb ached.

After many months of hospitalisation my son joined the family at the Mill. Our journey there was helped by an amazing inspiring social worker, Maggie, who kept me from sinking. I felt an overwhelming sense of relief and gratitude and was humbled by their enveloping care and concern.

My son, despite his severe difficulties, flourished in their care and is proud to have been part of the Mill. It gave him back his self esteem and coping mechanisms.

Nine months later another bombshell hits our family; his twin brother is struck by symptoms similar to his brother. Paranoia, fear, disasters occurring all around him. He being the saviour. At first I was in denial and the medical profession not convinced. Maybe he was attention seeking, mirroring, but, whatever, he was very disturbed and suffering deeply. Eventually he was sectioned after weeks of torment. More months of visiting hospital, sometimes nightmare visits. My organisation skills had to reach another level. I had work, the rest of the family, my two sons in pain.

My second son also spent many months at the Mill after hospital. They will both remember those days as the happiest days of their lives, being embraced by love, understanding, humour and common sense. They felt safe and were given hope which we all need a little of to survive. Indeed, more than that, everyone in the Mill thrived. The Mill is a legend, all who have passed through it are still 'family' to this day.

I have not talked about how my sons' illness manifested itself. I find the word 'illness' difficult. I try to find other words. The medical profession say schizophrenia, which I was told was a devastating diagnosis. At the onset one tries to justify and rationalise the bizarre thoughts and behaviour, searching for reasons. However, eventually I realised something inexplicable and frightening was happening. Worst of all it was completely out of my control. There was nothing I could do to make it better. My mother's instincts were useless, my umbilical cord scrambled.

The voices come and go but in stressful situations they are worse. It is very evident when they are there. Inappropriate behaviour, strange associations, paranoia. At the beginning, the presence of TV cameras everywhere, messages from the TV and radio, devastating tragedies here and everywhere, children addicted to heroin ("poppy kids" as one son called them). School teachers, heroin dealers, special powers, telepathy. Religion is a large part of their thoughts. They are instructed by God. Visitations from God, being God. Strange words, unintelligible at times. Feeling in danger, needing protection, under attack. People spiking their drinks is one of my son's obsessions. Feeling people out to kill them. One son asks for euthanasia constantly and talks of suicide. He has made several attempts. He jumped in the river at Green Quay, was admitted to Intensive Care after a very serious overdose, has tied things round his neck. The pain he is in is obvious, but I cannot really imagine the suffering. My pain in comparison must be nothing, but I do feel deep, deep pain and a feeling of helplessness. Just the other day he said "I'm going to call it a day; God has realised".
One of my sons, with time and medication, has improved beyond all measure and has a busy fulfilled life although the voices are never far away. He has learnt to deal with them and so have we as a family.

Sadly my other son is not better and struggles to survive. I now believe he is not able to survive in the community. It works for some but not all. I have no idea what the future holds for him and at times I despair, for there are very few other options.

Prejudice and stigma still exist, but there are also some wonderful individuals out there who are caring and understanding, not judging. However, we are running out of public places, pubs and restaurants, to go, having beaten hasty exits or at worst been banned for what is perceived as disruptive behaviour. This usually happens at times of high emotion, Christmas, family holidays and celebrations etc. There has been involvement with the police and courts. People do not generally understand, as to all intents and purpose people with mental health problems look like everyone else. They are not in a wheelchair, have two arms, two legs, but inside their heads is a frightening world and social interaction can be hard.

On a positive note they are free thinkers, their thought processes and ideas not hindered by a sensor button.

Schizophrenia is the "label" given to them and their lives, now the lives of their family and friends will be the same, it affects everyone. My family and friends have now accepted the change and up to a point have learned to deal with it. We have been supported by so many friends and health workers, too numerous to mention, and I would hate to leave anyone out. I acknowledge how their love and support have helped and we are indeed blessed. My partner has stuck with me through thick and thin and I truly thank him.

Coping with schizophrenia in the community as a mother is like being in the wilderness or at times on the front line without a gun. Where others can walk away I cannot and never will, but I am not prepared to sacrifice my life completely and realise I deserve a life too.

Balancing all that is a work of art, but I need to remain strong to cope.

There are dedicated caring individuals working in the community, but the system is flawed, there are not enough resources or safe places. There are some people who fall through the net and there are not enough respite beds. The nature of the condition renders them liable to be outcast from society, excluded, facing hostility. Under threat of eviction from social housing if they do not keep up the standards imposed. Facing B & B's, night shelters, strained family accommodation already at breaking point, and, the worst scenario, living on the street. A wave of fear hanging over them is exacerbating their paranoia. Hospital admissions are discouraged even if they have proven to be a danger to themselves or the community.

Expectations from a few professionals are unrealistic, imposing their own standards and values. I have felt anger and frustration from these expectations, just longing for them to be able to achieve them. They too have dreams, a rewarding job, children, someone to love, peace, a good night's sleep, and success.

At times I have felt I am to blame, if their so called behaviour has occurred. In the minds of some I receive the same hostility, condemnation and rejection. Now I am sounding paranoid!

Hopefully one day research will come up with an answer. Our family has been part of a research study at the Institute of Psychiatry.

The journey we have been through has at times been heartbreaking, but there has been laughter as well as tears and you could say life has not been boring. You play your hand with the cards you are dealt. Life does go on and everything is possible in a different way. There is so much more to write, but one of the side effects of supporting a family in the community is exhaustion, but I have tried to do my best.

"It ain't easy" for any family dealing with mental health issues but most of all let them know you love them.

"There are lanterns of life around to shed light in the darkness". (Adrian Mitchell)

I dedicate this piece of rambling to the Mill and all involved with it. Dave and Helen, you planted a beautiful seed.

As a final note some inspiring words from the American Poet, Maya Angelou.

"The issue is not how to survive, because obviously we are already doing that, somehow. The issue is how to thrive with some passion, some compassion, some humour and some style. I hope we can do that.

As I write this my second son is at the Mill for two weeks in the 'alternative to hospital' bed. His twin brother is very envious.

In conclusion this poignant, sad, courageous and sometimes humorous collection of memories and experiences are inspirational. Many of the residents from the Mill and sister houses undertook challenging journeys. However, under the gentle persuasion, guidance and encouragement from Dave, Helen and their dedicated team went on to realise their own potential.

Sadly, some fell by the wayside when out on their own in their own world. Indeed, my son was one near casualty. As changes in criteria for finding such safe houses altered, placements were hard to achieve. Changes in health and safety policies, new regulations, no smoking policies had an impact on family run homes, which offered comfort and solace to the vulnerable. More and more people were coping in B & B's, flats, hostels, in unsuitable environments without adequate support.

Sometimes the challenge was too great and my son was one who tried to end the pain by jumping from a 3rd floor window, narrowly escaping death or permanent serious disability. It was only this that highlighted the need for more intensive support which he is now receiving thanks to the intervention of some dedicated professionals.

Dave and Helen set the foundations for mental health care in this area and ran their houses as flagships to aspire to. Without them provisions in the King's Lynn area would be even more barren and desperate.

Despite well deserved retirement, nothing stops Dave and Helen's enthusiastic commitment to their beliefs and philosophies. They continue to fund raise and help those in need. Their compassion is tinged with humour and to receive it is like basking in the sunshine with a good glass of red wine.

Let's raise our glasses to a great achievement; The Millers' Tales.

Thank goodness Dave and Helen had the vision to follow their dream.

CHAPTER FOUR

In our early years I would try to get my interventions with people right. On reflection, at times I was ridiculous and unrealistic. Probably one of my biggest overactive rescuing of one young woman was this. Panic attacks, hyperventilating, obsessions, cleanliness anxiety, eating disorder – you name it, this lady had it – I don't mean to be unkind, that's just how it was. Sleeping was a problem. She felt unsafe on her own and her anxiety was at its worst at night. I thought a good night's sleep would do her the power of good, but the only way I could think of this happening was to offer to stay in her room. I set the Z bed up and we settled to sleep for the night, my bed close to hers to create the safety she required. As always, my head hits the pillow and I'm snoring, undisturbed till the morning. I was only asleep for a short while when her foot pushed me awake. I held a paper bag to her face until her breathing returned to normal as she had been hyperventilating. She was clearly disappointed in me. I suggested that I sleep in the bottom end of her bed to increase her security. I woke up at 7.30 to find the bed empty. I wandered downstairs. The young woman was drinking coffee and looked at me with dissatisfaction. I said I was sorry and asked her why she didn't wake me. She said she had tried. Another panic attack had come on, she tried pushing and kicking me but apparently I was in a star fish shape, taking up most of her bed, and didn't stir. I'm afraid I'm like my mother – we used to have to sit her up and shake her. I look back now and think, whatever was I trying to do? I couldn't rescue every situation. I learnt so much along the way and I hope that this book reflects this.

My mum never really seemed to know what my job entailed. I don't think she ever really thought it was a job. My Aunt told me that when they were together on holiday, my mum would tell the other holiday makers about her children's professions. "Paul is a doctor, Rosheen is a nurse, Philip works around the world for a big company." As an afterthought mum would say that "Helen has a home for people with problems." She was very proud of all of us but just found it difficult to describe what I did.

I feel that my mum and I shared a lot of the same characteristics and although we didn't argue, at times we would irritate each other. I look back and wish I had put more effort into our relationship. Mum died of cancer when she was 77. Philip, Paul, Rosheen and I were all with her when she died at home. We all cried together and felt very close. I wish I had told her how lucky I felt having such a fantastic family and how much I loved her and dad. I never really felt grown up enough and would look at her faults rather than all the positive things she gave us all. At the Mill when people moaned about each other or their own families, I would tell them to look at others' positive characteristics, believing that there are always good things you can find. I also used to say "Your mum and dad are the only ones you've got or are going to have, so try and accept them as they are; none of us are perfect".

For most people this message may have helped to forgive, forget and move on. For some, the pain of being the victim of abuse and torment was too great to leave behind. I'm sure for most people there are things in their life that they would change, or some regrets. Most of us have the odd skeleton in the cupboard. In fact I remember saying this to one of our favourite social workers called Jim one day. He was having woman problems. He said "Helen, I wouldn't mind the odd skeleton but I have a graveyard inside my cupboard". He did make me laugh.

Throughout my adult life I have had a real battle with my thoughts and feelings of getting pregnant at 16. I have always felt so ashamed of my irresponsible behaviour. Over the years I lied about my age and my boys' ages. If this book is published my age and pretence will be over. I feel it's good to own your demons.

I did feel so guilty that I had disgraced my parents. I can still remember the horror in their faces. They set me up to have an abortion but I walked out on the consultation with the Consultant and refused. I couldn't see what the problem was. I was madly in love with Michael. His parents bought our first home and I never look back with regrets of any of it. To this day I still struggle with how society can be your judge and jury. Of course it's not ideal and, yes, it's irresponsible to get pregnant so young, but it's not the end of the world and you can still achieve things and you can still cope. I have loved every minute of my children growing up and am so proud of all of them, and I'm sure they are of me. I'm sorry that I caused my parents so much shame and anxiety at that time. It's difficult for parents, sometimes. We judge ourselves too harshly. I am a firm believer that if good foundations have been built in early years most of us will be OK within life's rich tapestry.

I guess our philosophies developed over the years and became stronger as we learnt along the way. Initially we set out to help everyone increase his or her self-esteem and confidence, believing that these were the two major components people needed to be comfortable in their own skin. I suppose in the early days we wanted to rescue and save every individual who came through our front door. I saw very wounded and damaged people come through and I really wanted to make them all better. I've always had a very strong practical streak in me and so the emotional stuff really didn't last for long. I soon thought to myself; here we are today and where are we going to go tomorrow? People did tell me a lot about their lives and shared some of their most traumatic and deep secrets with me. I always told people that they had to concentrate on living for today and moving on to tomorrow. But, other than listening and just reassuring them that there was nothing they could do about some of the things they talked to me about, there was nothing else I could do. So we would look to do things that would really help build confidence and that were giving them lots of different experiences, such as having manners, respect, some fun, social graces, and some expectations. It was largely about learning to relive their lives again, with a lot of basic information that many of our residents didn't have. I'm not saying that they were unintelligent people, because some of our residents were extremely bright and intelligent. There were academic people, very skilled in some ways, but for some of the people coming through there was a basic lack of understanding of the world and social skills, practical skills and every other skill necessary really to be able to combat life. This was perhaps the time we really began to understand the corrosive impact of mental illness had on people's personalities, especially schizophrenia.

What is schizophrenia?

It is a mental disorder which affects thinking, feeling and behaviour. It is most likely to start between the ages of 15 to 35 and will affect about 1 in every 100 people during their lifetime.

Although the word 'schizophrenia' is often associated with violence in the media, this is the exception rather than the rule. Hospital admission is often not needed and many people with schizophrenia live a stable life, work, and have relationships.

What causes schizophrenia?

It seems to be a combination of different factors. These include genes, subtle brain damage at birth or viral infections during pregnancy and childhood abuse. Street drugs (ecstasy, LSD, amphetamines and crack) can probably trigger it and teenagers using cannabis can also be vulnerable. Stressful events and family tensions make it worse.

A good example of how complex the damage can be to the individual and those around them is illustrated by a young woman who came to the Mill with damaged thoughts and ideas. My initial reaction to her was one of a need to keep my distance because it felt that she needed to come to me as opposed to me reaching out to her. She presented as the "perfect teenager". She had a head turning physical appearance; long golden curly hair, a slight build, and bright sparkly eyes which held a distance to them. However, this belied what was going on inside. She has had an enormous impact on both myself and other staff as to how the mind can play cruel tricks in creating a life of confusion and distress. In a fair world this young woman would have been able to exercise her aptitude and ability and therefore choose her life's path that so many of us take for granted.

I have included the full version of her account she gave to me in her words and as you read it I would like you to imagine yourself in her shoes. Some of her language is obscure and where I have felt it helpful I have added my explanation in brackets.

What must it feel like knowing you are somebody else. You could read this next piece of work and feel confused; it may not make sense to you? It may be too far fetched for you to believe. The author of this piece of work is one of the most beautiful people you could hope to meet. She is very attractive and has above average intelligence, yet lives in a world of delusion. She feels that two famous people are her real brothers. She believes that one day they will come and find her and take her back to the 'real world' that she has been taken from. I know it sounds insane, but can you imagine believing whole heartedly in something that is not true and only you know the truth, yet cannot convince or change anybody's mind? We have had residents who think they are God or that they belong to the Royal family or that they are millionaires. Many residents have been left completely debilitated because of their obsessive delusional belief system. The young person who wants to be named as Flossy (that is what I have always called her) has kindly given me her story to share. Read it with belief and I think it will give you a journey into her everyday life. I have not been able to use her real name or the names of the famous people she believe to be her family. This was the condition of us sharing her story.

Flossy's Story:

As I write this, tears stream down my face. With every heartbeat my head and heart pound with an unbearable physical pain. I believe someone has taken my life without taking my breath; someone has stolen my identity. I do not know how and the funny thing is I don't know what my true identity is. Am I funny, am I clever? This life was cut short but should still be living. We try to identify with this forgotten life, we all try to show this shell of who I really am. We are as one but not completely. We have different beliefs, different strengths but I do believe that they are

showing me who I should have become.
I have such belief in my "should be" world that it makes it hard to breathe. I, or we, do not know how to live in this world. When I look in the mirror a person stares back at me. I do not recognise this person. I don't think I even look how I was supposed to look. I feel no connection with the image. A person stares back at me; sometimes I hesitate for I do not know her. It is not me. I look deep into the eyes, trying to stare through them and see if I can catch a glimpse of myself; the real me.

I feel like a ghost, my soul lost. In this world I am nobody; I do not exist, literally, for I do not belong here. I so know this to be true as much as I believe people have to breathe to stay alive. THEY took me away and killed me, leaving a shell. I can see, I can talk, I can laugh. I can believe I am happy, I can believe that I am alive but I do not live. (I do not know who 'they' are.)
I am alive when my heart and mind open and the realisations of my true path hit me. I live for the world in my head. I function automatically here, but with a purpose there, living out my real destiny, catching a glimpse of what life would have been like thus far, but what it will be like someday. When I can't go to this place, I feel lost, scared, lonely and hopeless.
I cannot live here; I know too much. I con myself into thinking that I have feelings but I do not. Apart from the communications everything is surface level. I do feel fear, anger and sadness. Fear that I will never live my life, anger that it has been taken away and sadness with the worry of never getting it back.

Nobody has ever understood the absolute intense feelings surrounding my real family. I am looked on as stupid. Because nobody believes me it makes me feel so deeply sad, hurt and completely alone. I sometimes can sort of understand but when people here [the Mill] people I like, and respect do not believe what I tell them about P and R it feels like they are denying ME, rejecting me. [P and R are famous personalities who this young women has identified as being her brothers. Regardless of how carefully it is explained to her that this is irrational she is unable to believe they are not her brothers].
I have never felt so strongly about anything. I know in my heart

that they are my destiny, like a loving mother knows she would give her life for her child. It is without question the one true belief that I have ever held.

Without P and R my heart breaks and my head shatters. The feelings I have for them are like a tidal wave, an earthquake, the end of the earth. I believe it to be love. I love so much I could die instantly; would this make my world right again? I cannot be certain, for at times my shell gets confused with me. Do I love? - I love my life as it should have been and the people I know in spirit and mind but not again physically (yet). Do I live? - we live separate identities, swimming in the shell reaching for the same purpose and the same people. These people are separate but joined; joined by hurt, pain and things that should have been - so nearly been. Separated by time, places, beliefs. They tell me(?) who I am supposed to be.

I criticise the shell at times for being useless, for not trying to live like those I have met on the wrong path. It's as though if I can't make it in my world then my shell should try and make it in its shell. In my heart, however, I believe we can do no more than what there is already. I will not betray my true destiny or my rightful loved ones. I will be forever waiting for them to get me. I so believe this will happen; if I didn't then I would terminate the shell.

I will love but not here
I will live but not here
I will be but not here

Well, not in the way a person is supposed to love, anyway. I think I do feel love here; it was perhaps the biggest gift P and R gave me before I was taken. [This refers to her natural parents who she believes took her from P and R.] I do feel guilty though. The fear here is indescribable. I want to love, I think, but I am scared it will be taken away.
I do not contribute to this society, not only because I feel guilty but because I don't know how to. I never learnt the lessons children learn as they grow. Maybe I rejected any lesson but I

am not so sure; basically there were no lessons, not from those physically around me anyway. I did learn from books and television. Before I realized P and R, I would transport myself into the TV and live with those on the screen, literally becoming part of the story. Only when the TV was turned off I was still there, in places I sometimes still visit.

I get increasingly agitated by people. Please don't get me wrong; these people I am dearly fond of, but I am not supposed to know them. Sometimes I almost don't want to know them for fear of becoming somebody different, somebody alien, and denying my true life. People here see me as a bad person I'm sure and I don't blame them. The communications I receive mirror the things that I believe people are saying and thinking. It is a constant battle; I so want to be a good person but I know I have done wrong. They tell me I am going to hell and I sometimes shed a tear knowing that they are right. I am so scared about this eventuality. [These communications are imaginary but completely real to her and not comments made by real people in contact with her. Despite constant reassurance that these are constructs of her mind she remains unable to sustain a belief that this is really the case.]

But for now, people around the shell and people inside __me__ help to ease the pain. When I look into P's eyes I see his soul - this is because I have always seen it, I have always been a part of it, and he part of mine. It's the worst feeling in the world, not being able to tell them both how much they mean to me. But I cannot communicate with them, only them with me. I need them to know that they are my spirit and I will forever await my return to them. It's not my fault that they are famous. I had them when they weren't in the public eye. It is lucky that they are because they are the key to my other life, but it is sometimes harder because people don't believe what I say about them. If they were 'ordinary' I am sure people would react completely differently.

They are close but at the same time so far. I cannot reach them with this faceless shell. People get in the way. There will come a time when none of this matters. The planets will align, the earth will shatter, and the bad people will have no voice. These bad people have stolen my life, my story (especially because of the TV programme). I cannot help but feel scared knowing that my hopes and dreams of a new, secure reality have been stolen, dangled in front of me and then shot to pieces intentionally.

CHAPTER FIVE

In the early days of the Mill there was a straightforward referral process to us from professionals such as Probation Officers, Social Workers, the Youth Offending Team, and housing and psychiatric consultants. It was a simple process to refer an individual because we had clear lines of communication and funding was quickly set up by the referring agency from money allocated to Social Services overseen by an appropriate manager. As time went on this changed. It is my belief that the advent of computers was a major factor in this by allowing managers to have access to a large data base, and economic factors began to take precedent over relevant care needs. Due to budgetary constraints set by the Government, managers were required to put greater emphasis on "value for money" and so, in my opinion, care for people with mental health issues began to deteriorate. This became evident by the referral process becoming more complex year on year, resulting in less of a mix of people. When referrals came from individual professionals it provided us with a rich mix of different personalities and backgrounds. This was more likely to provide a mix within the population of the Mill where less able individuals could model their behaviour on others more capable and in control of their own behaviour. Thus we had an atmosphere within the Mill of self support within the residential group. The referral process became the responsibility of various professions who would have to provide financial justification for their referral to a panel of managers at County level. This required that potential referrals had to meet specific criteria to qualify for funding. Because funding from the Government was always being cut back it led to a system based on the need to 'tick boxes'.

It is also my heartfelt opinion from years of first hand experience that individual professionals had to answer to their managers whose first priority was either financial or 'back covering'. If I had a pound for every time I heard someone say that I would be rich! This eventually led to those who shouted the loudest or whose client's behaviour became so outrageous or dangerous to the public that there was little choice other than supported accommodation. It was therefore inevitable that we ended up with people so damaged and similar in their illnesses that little modelling was possible. As the book unfolds there will be many examples of the system sadly failing people.

And so in the first few years of running the Mill, although people had quite complicated difficulties, there was a good mixture as opposed to those we encountered on the latter part of our Mill journey. Initially, we had people with depression. For instance, we had a woman whose four-year-old daughter had died of cancer and her husband then went off with somebody else which compounded her depression even further. Short term care was needed to help her over this very difficult time.

We had kids who had been abandoned and left care not knowing where to turn or what to do and got into trouble involving the police.

Because there were so many individual needs and different people I guess that was really one of the exciting things about our work. We had school teachers, professional writers and people who could barely read or write who had lived in care. Although it was expected that professionals would assess our homes for suitable placements, needless to say on one occasion our formal plan didn't work. I appreciate friends and families can become desperate in not knowing what to do for the best for their loved ones, particularly when they feel that there is a mire to get through before help is at hand. A local businessman rang up one day and asked us to assess his brother who had returned from travelling abroad and appeared not to be mentally very well. I invited them in for coffee and a chat. It was not long before the older brother asked if he could leave Tom with us and nip to town on some business. I thought it was a bit of a cheek but agreed. It would give Tom a chance to get a natural feel of the place and for us to get a feel for him and his needs. He was very quiet and withdrawn. Conversation was nonexistent; his eyes were dark and suspicious. Before we accept any resident we expected a full history report and several visits and a proper assessment to take place. This visit was supposedly to have an informal cup of tea, a snapshot look at how we operated and an introduction to each other. It was not unusual for us to have potential future residents visit. But on this occasion, hour by hour passed and nobody returned for him. We offered lunch, dinner, snacks, but nothing was accepted. Tom looked like a rabbit caught in the headlights. Nobody came back to collect him. We were as kind to him as we could be. We had all been duped. I made a bed for him in the spare room and told him we would get things sorted out in the morning. The family never returned and he was not known to any of the local psychiatric services. He refused to see a GP or any doctor and we had no funding or back up plan. We decided that we would try to engage with him over the next few days, which then turned into weeks. He was not able to be sectioned under the Mental Health Act because his behavior was not deemed to be of danger to himself or others. There was no history recorded to suggest otherwise. He had uncomfortable and strange behaviour patterns. He would sit for hours in the dark on the stairs. He would accept little food and not come out of his room for days. He would not engage with any of us. We didn't know if we or the children were safe. He was a completely unknown quantity. We decided in the end that we would take him to a bed and breakfast in King's Lynn and pay for him to stay for a few days. We told him that he would have to sort himself out from then on. He was a bright chap and capable of sorting benefits out for himself. We tried very hard to engage and befriend this lost soul but sometimes you haven't got what it takes and we felt we didn't have it. The decision was hard but there was nothing we could do, it was a no win situation.

All shapes and sizes and backgrounds merged inside Mill House. Ro, a private guest, arrived with her husband from their Norfolk holiday cottage. He was a company director from a well known international company. His wife had been in the medical profession but had long since retired. The expectations to wine, dine and be the company director's wife had all become too much and she had sought solace in alcohol. It was decided that a short break at our house would be beneficial to all the family.

And so a very well spoken, slight woman arrived with her Gucci handbag and case. We had not been told that her main problem was alcohol dependency – that could have explained why her bags were so heavy. Residents often arrived with a black bin bag or a few Tesco carrier bags. As the extent of her alcohol problems unravelled she would relate many amusing stories that would have us rolling with laughter. She was quite a character to say the least. On one occasion at her son's school the Head teacher had been alerted by the caretaker that a parent had been spotted lurking in the bushes making sure her son was all right. The parent in question was Ro. She was escorted off the premises, and her husband was called to collect her because she was drunk in charge of her 'Jag'. She was eventually banned from the school.

On another occasion she was asked to leave a corporate dinner function after becoming too exuberant in conversation with important business contacts. It was suggested by his fellow Directors that it might be better if she was left at home in future.

After a short while of her residing at The Mill, divorce papers were served and child protection became an issue as her husband felt it was inappropriate for her to be alone with their child.

He refused to provide her with any money for her personal needs and ceased contact. Her need for booze was an incessant craving; at times she would drink anything that had an alcoholic content in it, however small. Once she stole Dave's cough mixture. He was less than impressed as he thought he was seriously unwell. Normally Dave was well mannered and calm but not on that occasion.

Ro decided a trip to the Department of Social Security was essential in order to obtain some money for her everyday needs – her fees were being paid direct to us from her husband. Ro was a very bright articulate woman who did not take no for an answer easily. After being told that she was not entitled to any financial support, she calmly asked if she could use their toilet before she left the DSS office. The key was given to her, and after thirty minutes of her not returning the it, security was sent for. Yes, she was still in the toilet demanding a cheque be posted under the door before she would leave the building. It was now

5.00pm and they wanted to close. I received the call and set off to persuade Ro to come out of the toilet.

One day we had a visit from "Mr Jobsworth' our local policeman, who asked if he could search the room of a young man who was staying with us. Not wanting to offend, I agreed. When he came downstairs, I asked him what he was looking for. He said "A sack and some garden shears". I started to feel myself getting hot and feeling 'duped'. I asked why he thought a young 18 year old, who was very smart and trendy, would want such things. He said he had been told about "places" like ours and what sort of people lived in them. Ro was privy to this conversation. He also said he nearly purchased the house opposite but pulled out when he realised that we lived across the road. He was rude and arrogant. Ro in her posh voice, speaking the Queen's English, confronted him about his attitude, told him who she was and that she would be reporting him to his superiors. He was a pig! I just lost my temper, told him to f*** off out of our house. As I physically pushed him along he was threatening me with prosecution. Ro and I pushed the large front door closed once he was over the threshold.

Ro decided to return to her holiday cottage after living with us, once her finances had been sorted. Over the period she had been with us we had taken her to hospital when unconscious from booze and sat with her when she was hallucinating, something we both found terrifying. I also forgave her for drinking my entire home made wine stock that I had collected for many years. We used to have lots of parties at the Mill and I had stored this wine in large demijohns on shelves in a cupboard upstairs. When we were having one of our parties I collected some of the demijohns and was delighted to see how clear the wine was. However, on tasting the wine I discovered every demijohn contained weak tea. I was deeply shocked and surprised at the depths her addiction had driven her to. I can't believe to this day how naïve I was. The demijohns used to look handsome on their big wooden shelves in the kitchen and the store cupboard upstairs – inside her bedroom; we live and learn.
It was then we realised we were not able to provide the specialist

care needed for people with alcohol dependency. However, life is not that clear cut.

A Social Worker by the name of Adrian worked closely with us and said he knew of a man who desperately needed the type of support we could offer. This man's name was James. He was alcohol dependant and living rough. Adrian believed that it would not be long before he died because he was so deeply into his dependency. James was currently in hospital 'drying out' and Adrian believed it was now or never for James. James did come to the Mill and tells his story;

My name is James Munroe and I was born in Sheringham, a small sea fishing town.   I lived with Mum and Dad and my brother and sister.   I enjoyed a happy childhood with gentle parents who were the 'salt of the earth'.   Life was full of adventure, surfing and lazing on the beach.   I really got into my music and as I got older I started playing in local bands and became well known in Sheringham for my guitar playing and impersonations.   I was banned from the pub for a week after pretending to be an Aphid and gobbling up all the plants.   I also used to ride old fashioned bicycles through town wearing a top hat with a rear light strapped to my head.   "Here come the Red Arrows" I would shout riding through the pub and out the back door – they loved that one.

I worked as a gardener for Sheringham council and would see to the golf course and gardens which I really enjoyed.

Depression started to infiltrate my life. I started boozing heavily and leaned on alcohol.   Eventually I lost my job and home.   I had nowhere to live and spent my life living in the woods, friends' sheds and eventually set up a tent on the allotments.

One night a piece of tin sheeting came straight through the top of my tent.   It was raining heavily and I got soaked.

Temperatures at times would plummet and I would spend hours freezing in the cold.   I collected food from dustbins and at times the fish and chip shop would give me a free meal.   People were kind and looked out for me.   I was given slops that came out of the drip trays in the pubs as my addiction to booze had taken a firm hold.   One day I returned to the allotment to find that the bulldozers had been in. My possessions had been left in black bin bags. I repaired my tent using bits of lino and old carpet. I moved into the woods and was there for a few months.

My mental health deteriorated and soon I was to be rescued by a kind neighbour called Adrian Farncome. He was a social worker and he convinced me to go into the David Rice psychiatric hospital where I stayed for the next nine months. On leaving the David Rice I moved into the Mill House.

There were a few hiccups at first. I ran off with the fees money (money which is deposited in your bank when you first arrive for your care, which you hand in to staff) and went on a bender. I ended up in Sheringham and Helen and Dave had to pick me up as I was conked out on a bench at the railway station. I'd had a lot of money and was left with tuppence! They brought me back to the Mill and gave me a good talking to. Chances had been given, and if I didn't start to make an effort I would be out. In January 1991 I gave up drinking and have not had one drink since. I feel very lucky as so many people go back to it.

I started to do some repair work to keep my mind occupied. I am good with my hands. I was very shaky at first and had to take it a day at a time and my nerves and depression were still bad. I managed to get a workshop in the garden and Helen and Dave brought some tools and I was soon repairing Hoovers etc. and putting up shelves.

I met Lorraine at the Mill. We both loved the chickens in the garden and made them a chicken run. One chicken was called 'Mr Cockerel' and he would sit on my shoulder. Blast, I loved that chicken. We were offered some more chickens so we grabbed our torches and went down the road with a woman from the Mill to catch them. The police were informed because of the torches being shone in gardens and trees where the chickens were roosting. There were people running about and the police hot on our tail as they thought we were chicken rustling, but we'd been given permission to get them. I have never laughed so much in all my life.

A funny experience happened when we went for a day in Swaffham market. We went in the Mill minibus. It had a roof rack on which I piled high with bicycles and a station wheelbarrow I had purchased. Gwen was driving and she met us back at the bus and we were soon ready to go. We headed out of the car park gate and the bloomin' barrier hit the wheelbarrow and knocked it clean off. "What have you got on there?" Gwen said as the rack shot off the back. Len was in the bus and when I went to have a look I could hear him saying "That bloody boy". I got some wire to hold the rack on until we got home. We had to drive home with half the rack hanging off. Dave saw us as we arrived back at the Mill and said "What another load of old scrap; what the hell have you done to that rack?". Needless to say I had to repair that as well.

We used to go all over the place with the Mill. We had holidays and trips out. We would go to Fakenham where Helen would go on a shopping spree, usually buying some old stuff she set her eyes on. One day she brought so many pots that everybody had to ride home with them on their laps and by their feet; they were everywhere. She would sit in the front and stuff raw fish down her mouth which some said made them feel sick to see it, but that was just Helen!

Drink and Drugs:

I can only tell you from my opinion how detrimental drugs and alcohol can be. I have hung onto the toilet seat pan vomiting like most young people. I have been only too happy to smoke the weed as well. To me it was like inhaling garden herbs. I could see no harm. We live and learn. Friends to this day still enjoy a smoke and at one time I would be the first to roll. "They tell me it's good for you, it's relaxing, it's great to 'chill out'." "I can't see how it does anybody any harm." Well I have seen it on many occasions and it can do harm to some people. Would Julian ever have hanged himself if he hadn't found cannabis? I don't know. It does seem that many young people we have worked with have exacerbated their mental illness by excessive use of cannabis - or have they taken cannabis to help them feel more relaxed? Were they already having symptoms? It could be a chicken and egg situation. Do younger people move on to stronger drugs in the hope that it will block the torture already in their heads? Two deaths spring to mind; Sarah Pye and Peter Prior. Both of these young, talented people died as a result of a lethal heroin overdose. In my opinion, neither of these people wanted death as their outcome but the torment in their heads led to their actions in the hope of finding some peace.

Peter came to us for 'rehab' and support as his mental health was deteriorating fast. Peter soon settled in and it was not long before his love of music returned.

Peter earned money to have guitar lessons with a tutor named Andy Graham who recognised in him a real talent and worked with him for about a year. Peter played at 'The Crown' (the local pub) and at music nights in the 'Ffolkes Arms' and would attract a loyal and very proud following from friends, fellow residents and staff wherever he played.

Peter became close to Andy's sons, particularly Luke, and they would spend a great deal of time together jamming, with Peter playing a major role in Luke's early musical development. Peter would often visit Luke and pass on to him what he had himself learned during his lessons. Luke has now become a skilful and successful musician and Peter certainly played a part in this.

In time Peter left the Mill and married and had a baby daughter of whom he was immensely proud. He would visit the homes with her and seemed happy to be a family man. Sadly, however, Peter's troubles led to a premature death. Sadly Peter became very mentally unwell. He had used drugs in the past but had not touched them for a long period of time. Before he died Peter's mother had tried in vain to get professional help for Peter who was struggling with voices and tortured thoughts. He died of a heroin overdose. He is remembered with fondness and respect by all whose lives he touched including Sal, our charismatic 'gap' student who herself left memories behind for everyone she met. She tells us her story about how she viewed Peter (this made Dave cry);

The year I spent living with the Mill House was truly amazing, and one that will influence my life forever. Whilst that sounds so clichéd, there really isn't any other way to put it.

It was the people that made the time so special, and one person in particular who touched me deeply, and who will stay with me forever, was the beautiful Pete Prior.

Sitting on the back porch of this city share house, in Melbourne Australia, I am finding it hard to recall the detail of Pete's background to share with you, to provide you with a complete picture of this beautiful soul. However, what keeps coming to my mind more lucidly than any other memory are flashes of his gorgeous smile. A big unassuming, warm smile, interchanged with the occasional youthful shy-guy grin. That smile has always stayed with me.

Pete faced inner battles and the actions that stemmed from these sometimes confused and frustrated those around him, especially those that he loved. However, for people that knew him it wasn't hard to see Pete for who he really was; a truly beautiful compassionate soul, with an unmistakable gentle innocence about him.

I will always remember the first time I met Pete. Amelia and I had just arrived at the Mill House and Helen was giving us a quick verbal introduction in the Gap student cottage, our new home. I remember Pete walking around outside, subtly attempting to get a glimpse of us through the cottage windows. With an excited beaming smile, the first thing he asked me was if I played the guitar. Before long he was teaching me the rhythm guitar section to Jimi Hendrix's 'Little Wing' so Pete could play along doing the lead guitar. Pete would play Hendrix CD's on repeat and learn Jimi's riffs, bit for bit, and then play them for me, making it look so easy, with his hands effortlessly gliding around the frets, and often ending a piece with that honest coy like grin saying something like "But I'm still working on it... it's nothing like how Jimi played it".

Over the years I have played in a number of bands with many *talented and hard working guitarists and musicians, but I truly believe I will never get to play with someone as musically enthusiastic and naturally talented as Pete. I remember going on a trip to Edinburgh for a short holiday. Before I left I gave Pete a Waifs CD (my favourite Australian Folk Roots band at the time). I said "The guitarist in this band – Josh – is amazing, while I am away maybe you can learn a solo off <u>one</u> of the songs". When I returned a few weeks later, Pete had learnt just about every solo of every song on that album and could play them with as much presence and subtlety as was on the recordings!*

The owner of a big heart, Pete was a 'softy' and 'a gorgeous guy'. With a large sprinkling of Bruce Springsteen-like looks and charm, Pete was playful and at times cheeky. And whilst Pete was one of the youngest residents in the Mill House he also displayed a presence of mind beyond his years. There were many times where I was inspired by a certain acceptance he showed to others and to the situations he found himself in. On many occasions Pete was a sure cure for my homesickness, a source of great comfort and companionship for me, a true friend. I remember Pete carrying with him an abundance of love and gentle courage; he was consistently honest with me and a beautiful listener, always eager to know about Australia and my friends and family at home.

When I knew Pete he yearned to live life independently and to the fullest. Ultimately he dreamt of becoming a professional musician. I heard he found a loving partner and was father to a beautiful child. Unfortunately his life was cut short, which is an indescribable loss to his family, the Mill House and the broader community. However, for me, and I am sure a similar story is held by many others, Pete still holds a strong presence in my life. His memory continually provides me with inspiration for my music and the influence he has had on my journey is something that I am always thankful for.

When Dave let me know about Pete's passing I wrote a couple of songs for Pete, one song called 'Coolbreeze' which I now perform at most shows with my band here in Australia. When we play it live I often dedicate the song to Pete or I picture him in my mind. I remember that smile, I am reminded of how lucky I am to be performing up on stage, and how Pete would have loved to have been up there, and the truth is – most of the time he is!

"Oh what a smile....I like the way you hold your guitar – And I like your accent. And the cool breeze, I don't like it on my face – But I don't mind it through my hair; I'm getting used to it".

Often when residents reached for drugs or they would reach for alcohol as this was another way of blocking out the uncomfortable and sometimes relentless torture and anxiety. Sadly alcohol and drugs would often compound the problems even further. I'm not saying people who are unwell shouldn't drink. I have seen it act as a real tonic to some people, increasing their 'Dutch courage' and confidence. Most of us enjoy a social drink. I look forward to my glass of sherry on a Sunday when cooking the dinner and the kitchen becomes chaotic. I am such a 'lightweight'!
However, we were normally very cautious when taking a referral into any of the houses with a drink or drug dependency as their main problem. I feel that it is specialized work. Rehab with a tight structural regime was usually more suitable, although we did have some people do very well with us; as I said earlier, we can't always place people in boxes. We are unique and as individuals need our own package to identify our needs and to gain the necessary support for our future wellbeing.

Taking my early experiences of riding and using it in my working life at the Mill has been very enjoyable. We had a young lad of seventeen move in. I'll call him Mr H. He didn't want to come to the Mill but his life was being dictated by taking drugs in order to self medicate his mental health problems. He told me that drugs made him feel alive and gave him adrenaline. I taught him to ride over several months and each day he would help me feed, water and help with the normal duties of looking after a horse. The problem in the early days was that I only had one horse, so soon after, I advertised for a loan horse so that we could ride together. Mr H was keen and motivated and after a few months was riding well. We had another conversation about drugs - the only thing that seemed to excite him. I took him out for a ride and on reaching a large space of flat ground asked him to race me. Both horses went like the clappers and at the end of our gallop I could see beads of sweat on his forehead, his colour an extreme white. I asked him how he felt on the adrenaline front and he said that it was as good as taking drugs. I had made my point!

CHAPTER SIX

Working with other organisations was not always easy. However, our local doctors' surgery was exceptional in the service they offered The Mill House. Everyone was patiently listened to and nothing was too much trouble. There was a good working relationship between surgery staff and the Mill, even to the point of home visits by GPs. Occasionally an individual felt too frightened or anxious to attend the surgery and it was wonderful that this was understood. The same went for their pharmacy in terms of quickly making up prescriptions and being so cooperative. The same applied to Social Services. The Homes Registration Authority in particular worked closely with us, helping to develop our service to a high standard of care, providing training, guidance and support in a very respectful way. Silas, one of our Homes Registration Officers, was exceptional in his guidance. There were so many amazing professionals in our early years of working. There were consultants who would come out after hours to help if there was a problem. We felt that we were an important part of a team all shooting at the same goal which was the recovery of every resident. They would often give us their home phone numbers knowing we would not abuse it.

One of the most significant people we encountered along our Mill and Community Support Homes journey was Adrian Farncombe, a Social Worker whose role was placing clients back into the community for rehabilitation. He listened, supported us and his clients and was an inspiration and a role model to us all. One of our town houses is named after him; we called it Adrian Lodge. Sadly, Adrian died of cancer.

If Adrian suggested we give a particular client a chance and new beginning we would trust his judgement. This applied to the most complicated and colourful people. He achieved this by having faith in people and an instinctive sense in selecting the appropriate residents. However, on one occasion we did say no.

I also had a sixth sense and relied greatly on my intuition. The young person in question had impersonated doctors, had serious delusions about who he was, had been involved in stitching someone up in casualty and had been involved in many areas of theft and deception. He was very tall, very handsome and could 'charm the birds out of the trees'. I don't know why I said no, I just had a gut feeling. My 'Mother Nature' instincts just told me he was not suitable for us. I held firm on my decision even though staff and residents wanted to welcome him in. A few years later I picked up a national newspaper to find a full page article about the person in question. He had taken people's identities; impersonated doctors and surgeons and had been involved in many operations including removing a patient's appendix. He had been sentenced to indefinite hospitalisation in a secure unit.

Throughout our working years our local secure unit continued to offer an exceptional service. Over the years the roles of social workers, community psychiatric nurses and nurses were merged into one confusing organisation called The Community Mental Health Team (C.M.H.T.).

There was once a clear distinction between the roles of each profession. It seemed that overnight C.P.N.s had become social workers, having to fight for funding for anyone they deemed fit to go into residential care. In my opinion most workers seemed to have no idea of what they needed to do. There was an expectation that nurses and CPNs became 'acting Social Workers' but without the relevant experience with which to make appropriate decisions relating to their clients. I'm not saying they didn't do their job well, only that their experience was limited to their individual roles for which they had been trained. They were required to understand benefit systems and housing and financial issues and I felt they were 'working in the dark'. The support system no longer seemed to be working on the same side as us or the client. We had no choice but to work with some of the professionals as they were assigned to some of our residents. Some showed no respect to us or the client. It was as if there were very few 'good guys' left; the system seemed to 'grind' the good workers out of it. A CPN from Heacham who was a kind and empathetic worker left because his own mental health was suffering from working in the system. The clients he could cope with, the management he couldn't. He said his life had been made too difficult. In future years I was to meet many more professionals with a similar story who now sadly no longer work in the system.

It's hard for me to put pen to paper and explain my anger at how the system had become. I will give readers a flavour of what I mean. I won't be using names, and if I did they would perhaps deny all and this was a large part of the problem so only extracts can be used. I left the graveside of an ex resident after a small, harrowing service where I had read the heartfelt words that his loving wife had written. I felt that he should have been safely hospitalised under a section of the Mental Health Act, but he was now in the local graveyard after jumping in front of a car. Before this he had tried electrocuting himself and stabbing himself. This was after he had been released from hospital having taken a massive overdose. Two mental health workers followed Dave and me from the grave. They said to us that he didn't really want to kill himself and that he had pushed his attention seeking too far! I don't know if they ever told the driver of the car, who I knew personally. Gary, the driver and his wife June tell their story later in the book. Attention seeking behaviour remains a popular term used to avoid any responsibility by some 'professionals' involved in managing their clients' care. In my opinion the peaks and troughs of Eddie's behaviour clearly warranted the professionals taking much more of a proactive role which may have avoided his death. As far as I am concerned the question remains; should he have been sectioned under the Mental Health Act in order to keep him safe and protect others from his erratic and disturbed behaviour? At times there was a lack of care and respect within the teams of professionals, as illustrated by an anecdote related to me by a professional worker who was a friend of mine. She looked at me with hopelessness in her eyes. She said she was working on her computer one day when a Manager tapped her on the shoulder and said "Are you the worker for...?" She replied that she was and asked why. The manager said abruptly that this person had committed suicide and to make sure her notes were up to date. That was it! My friend was left devastated. I would say this was typical of how poorly staff were looked after in the system. Patients, residents and clients didn't stand a chance when faced with such uncaring attitudes from management.

A local CPN visited the Mill one day and vociferously complained to Nancy, one of our staff, that she had been waiting at the office and nobody had seen her. That was because nobody was in the office; something I was always pleased about. If staff were always in the office doing the 'mundane stuff' they were not out on the floor working and engaging with the residents - isn't that what was supposed to happen? This person was giving Nancy a really hard time about how much work she had to do and how much time she had wasted. Nancy pointed out a number of options that had available to her and how simply she could have found staff; i.e. ask a resident, walk through to the main house (we were not a locked unit). I listened for a while to her tirade until I could listen no more. I swung my chair around and asked her to leave the premises. The same woman was a key worker for another resident. She had done her upmost to move this person out into independent living; something which had already been tried and failed. She lied about the input she had given this person, and in one review, a member of our staff and the resident were left open mouthed. They were not confident enough to say anything as they both feared the consequences. This worker manipulated another resident into moving house rather than working through the problems she was having. We were told that under no circumstances were staff to make contact once she had moved as it would be too unsettling. She then transferred the case to a male colleague, the resident's worst nightmare. This resulted in an unnecessary move to the middle of nowhere. I kept waiting for news. The relationships between residents and staff were very often the only ones they had and such intervention irrevocably damaged this. It could be assumed that the resident could make contact with staff, but unfortunately some residents lack the confidence to speak out.

I have thought about why such a cavalier stance was taken by this CPN and believe it to be for a number of reasons; warped thinking, manipulation of facts, jealousy or getting even in some sick way. I do know it doesn't feel good. I am not in any way against people being moved for appropriate reasons to other homes; there were some very good Homes out there with more experience than we had. However, I do not believe the isolation of this particular home was not beneficial in this case. The home to which the resident moved was a great place, in fact we helped them set up in their early days as we did other local private resources. Competition and choice had never been a problem to us. It's healthy for a resident to have choice. But the moving of this resident, I felt, was based on a simple dislike for us and our organisation. At the time of writing the lady in question was being buried having been found dead in her independent flat which was under the care home umbrella.

On another occasion a resident called John was moved from our sister house. His initial diagnosis was high anxiety, depression and paranoia. His new Consultant and the professional team surrounding him were asked to make an assessment of this resident's mental health, as the Social Services budget had been overspent and they wanted to move him on. I have no doubt that yet again financial considerations had become the priority. No credit was given to comments from the staff about this very vulnerable man. We explained to Social Services that his wife had recently filed for divorce and had been caught sleeping with his friend in the room above his flat. He had also been hit by her new lover. He couldn't defend himself against a fly. He was bright and intelligent but emotionally disabled. The stress and anxiety which resulted from the breakdown of his marriage led to more and more bizarre behaviour. At times he was able to present as bright and intelligent and at others, when feeling lost and vulnerable, inappropriately put on children's and women's clothing. He was given a months' notice to leave his supported accommodation. His CPN was powerless and clearly felt very uneasy about the decision but had to 'watch his own back'. This was a catch phrase I became used to hearing and which eventually made me want to scream. The new system led to the application of a ruthless management power over both workers and clients.

In their wisdom they moved John to a hostel in Wisbech which was cheap and completely inappropriate. I decided one day to call by and take him out for a coffee. I was met by a cheerful member of staff who launched into all the reasons why she felt this man shouldn't be there. For instance, he was being exploited by others living there, who were mainly tough young men on bail or probation. 'Just great', I thought. I went in and knocked on his door and it took a few attempts before he would answer. I shouted through the door that it was Helen. He said "OK" and I heard him slide the furniture away from behind his locked door. He opened up and let me in. I was taken aback by what I saw. He was looking like a victim from a prisoner of war camp. His small room was a mess, he was unshaven and looked haunted. I was very casual in my approach and suggested he have a shave and clean himself up before going out for a bite to eat. He couldn't shave as he had no equipment. He couldn't change as he had no clean clothes. So he went out as he was. He never complained. His meek and mild personality didn't allow for this emotion. At the 'Bakers Oven' he ate and drank copious amounts. Slowly with my inquiring questions he told me that his pay day had been two days earlier and that he had been taken to the post office to collect it by one of the new house mates, who had then taken his money from him. He had no money for food but had told nobody. The care staff at the hostel said he never seemed to make himself food in the communal kitchen! He told me that the other house mates frightened him and therefore he only left his box room when necessary. I left him with money, food and a razor and organised for him to come and stay at the Mill House's guest bed for a break. In the car on my return to Kings Lynn, I cried with anger and frustration. How could this be okay? I reported my findings to the CPN who had his own personal difficulties together with problems with his management. As always his team were less than impressed by my interfering. They said I had a problem with letting go. I threatened to start a private court case which I would fund unless something was done. He was soon placed in a supported hostel back in Kings Lynn. Again the placement was insufficient support for him. This hostel had a good staff team and reputation and was set up to look after the mentally unwell and provide rehab. However, they soon found that his needs were beyond their remit despite their best efforts. His mental health had deteriorated and hospital admissions followed. Again, I asked if he could return to our sister house, only to be told no. He was moved into an old folk's home for he had now been diagnosed with dementia. I spoke to his CPN who said that his deterioration was because of natural causes and nothing could be done. He died of a heart attack shortly afterwards. I think he probably died of a broken heart and spirit. If dementia was his final destination, wouldn't it have been better for him to live at our sister house where he had been settled, content and accepted; somewhere where he was cared for and happy? We were paid under £2 an hour for his care. The hostel in Kings Lynn would not have been any cheaper, but it came out of a different budget than social services. I still feel so angry about the disgusting care he received. But oh no, it seems we must not challenge the professional decision makers! They know best. I wonder how many more such clients are out there in our caring system, or am I just being over protective?

Slowly but surely the mishmash of people over the years came through the door, and each and every one of them was an individual, but the same philosophy stood for everybody. There were a few basic rules, one of which was to respect each other and yourself and we would always strive to do that. We didn't employ cooks, cleaners or a gardener because we considered the Mill was our home, which meant we were all living together and there were responsibilities that went with that. Quite simply, if you didn't peel potatoes or prepare vegetables then we wouldn't eat. If we didn't clean the yard, mow the grass, keep the hedges cut and weed the garden well then it would all look a mess. If we didn't wash our clothes or ourselves then we would look unkempt. So basic functioning was part of our everyday life.

There was no getting up late in the day and going to bed late at night. People could go to bed whenever they wanted, but though not a rule, it was a subtle expectation that everybody would pitch in on the morning chores. If we were all going to participate in getting the house organised and cleaned up then we needed to be ready. This was aided by peer pressure from the residents and staff team. That meant people had to be disciplined in organising themselves. We would regularly join for cups of tea and a cigarette round the kitchen table. Every day we had fresh cooked food which was a really important event. I loved cooking and I certainly encouraged most of the residents to participate in learning how to cook; even if it was really basic food, I just felt everybody would benefit from a healthy diet.

We wouldn't have exotic food, instead we would have simple fare like fresh lasagne and salad, meat pudding, meat pie, pork chops and chicken. Every now and then we would have a food theme night, such as Chinese or Indian and residents would pick what they wanted to cook. They would make a list of ingredients, purchase them and create a meal. Those not directly involved in cooking would be responsible for creating an atmosphere by using relevant props such as wooden spoons and tin plates as musical instruments, low level tables and lighting. On these particular evenings everyone had fun singing and dancing – well, we would try to get everyone involved. At the Mill nothing was straightforward and despite our best efforts of inclusion we could never account for the exceptional level of creative excuses or beliefs that some residents held, preventing them from taking part. Such as a tight bra preventing a woman from washing up, or another woman who refused to turn up to her birthday celebrations because despite a resplendent spread being provided there were no chicken drumsticks on offer as had been the case at a previous resident's 21st! Dave did however try to appease the situation with a quick dash to Tesco, but the damage had been done!

I always feel that fresh air, exercise, and a bit of cooking are great therapies. There was strong encouragement to get up and participate. We also did a lot of outside activities like walking the dogs every day, or we would hop into the vehicle and go to Sandringham. At other times we would go for nice walks, picnics by a ford or the beach, swimming, go down to the sailing club, walk, have a swim and walk round the lake. I felt it was my responsibility to actively engage residents in outside pursuits as opposed to staring at walls.

CHAPTER SEVEN

Holidays were an annual part of the Mill life and would be anticipated and argued over with enthusiasm and vigour. No two people wanted to go to the same place and where some packed months in advance others could be found filling a black bin bag on the morning of departure, while still others were oblivious to the need for any luggage at all. For some the change of routine was too unsettling for them to participate. Others didn't want to holiday with the same people they lived with, although a new environment often transformed personalities. Holidays varied from day trips out to more challenging ventures overseas, the purpose being to widen horizons.
Join me on our trip to Ostend;

The map was drawn and placed on the sitting room wall. Residents, Dave and I had decided an opportunity for character building and adventure was a must for this particular year's house holiday. We had found a sailing boat funded by a charitable foundation. The challenge was to raise nearly £2,000 to take a gang of us to Bruges and Ostend. Together we cleaned cars, held jumble sales, bingo and musical events and raised the sum required. Our financial achievements were recorded on the sitting room wall and step by step our goal was achieved. Nine eager residents were chosen along with Dave, myself and our dear friend Dave Butterworth who was regularly recruited to help out on all of our ambitious trips away. Sailing experience between us was limited.

Our vessel was a 70 foot ketch moored at Ipswich. We spent the first day tacking up and down a river which is quite good fun, although one day was enough, as we all wanted to get to Belgium. The crew, a skipper, skipper's mate and two crew told us that everyone had to be able to swim. 'Whoops'; we did take young Sadie with us who had agoraphobia and had hardly stepped outside of Litcham village, let alone swim. We thought that anyone entering the North Sea probably wouldn't have any less of a chance than the rest of us, so she came along.

The skipper briefed us; there would be shifts of three hours each while sailing, continuing on that basis until the arrival at our destination. We divided up into three residents and one member of staff per shift (or watch as I think the nautical term is). I didn't like the skipper's attitude; he had a superior air about him and clearly was less than impressed with us as a gang. He spent much time in his cabin and at one point I heard him on the telephone to his lady friend talking about us in derogatory terms. His lady friend spent the night with him on the vessel, only leaving the next morning. I told Dave about the telephone conversation and the next day I confronted him. I told him that we were not a group of 'public school kids' and we were entitled to respect and if possible to reach the destination we had set ourselves...My card was marked! You don't ever question a skipper even if he is selfish, thoughtless, insensitive and in need of female company.

The skipper was not keen on doing the crossing to Ostend, that much was obvious, but our happy holiday makers were very keen. We learned that a gale was expected that night, but if everyone was willing and prepared to do the job we could go for it, so we motored out leaving at around 2am for the tide. Not far out the wind got up and we were sailing along nicely. The wind gets up a bit more and then even more, by which time it was running at a force 8 and the sea was very lively. And of course it was dark. Helming, you got a glimpse of a wave towering above you and then you were on top of it. We were licking along at what the skipper told us was 11 knots, ploughing up the crest, going so fast we would drop like a stone the other side, with a crunch and a crash and then it's up to the next wave and the same again and again. My stomach started rolling within the first few miles of our journey. Soon I had left behind my breakfast, dinner and tea of the day before and any morsel of food and drink I had taken in. Although the sea was exciting as we corkscrewed along, I had never felt so ill in all my life. I lay on the deck in the middle of the night on my watch, the rain and sea lashing down on top of me as I sat harnessed to the boat. One of the crew belonging to the boat suggested to the skipper I be taken off duty, explaining how unwell I was. Having woken him up, guess what he said – No, she must not leave her watch. There was no fight left in me. I didn't care if I lived or died, I was past caring and too weak to move. Someone woke Dave and he virtually carried me downstairs, undressed me, put me in warm clothes and into bed. He thought I had hypothermia and kept giving me sips of hot drinks. It sounds so dramatic but that's how it was. It was so unlike me as I'm usually the tough one.

The toilets or heads as they were called were in demand and the rules are straightforward; nothing but what comes out of you and toilet paper go in the toilet, which is then pumped out by hand through a macerator. There's always one, isn't there? She forgets this rule and flushes a pair of disposable pants, which promptly block up one of our toilets for the rest of the trip. There was a bit of poetic justice though, when she was sitting on the loo one time and failed to hear the shout that we were going to tack. One moment she's sitting on the loo with her back to the wall, the next the boat has shifted from 45 degrees one side to 45 degrees on the other. That little combination equals one person with their drawers round their ankles catapulting to the middle of the galley – oops!

On reaching Ostend everyone was eager to get going to find chocolate and good coffee. I could hardly walk and had no appetite. I staggered round like a drunk and was pleased to return to the boat to lie down. The skipper looked delighted about the state of me and announced that I would be in charge of cooking a roast dinner for everyone that evening. When I suggested that a small oven and two gas rings were not the ideal cooking companion for a roast dinner for sixteen he shouted at me and said I was to do as I was told. I nearly cried. I don't know if it was because I was so ill and he was being such a b...... to me or frustration of being shouted at in front of everybody. The dinner went well, with my grit and determination and my being pretty good in the kitchen. A couple of the gang helped me out.

DB remembers more of the journey home than I do:

The return journey was a direct crossing in daylight for most of the way and in fine sunshine. We were buzzed by a Belgian air force plane presumably checking us out and arrived outside Felixstowe by nightfall. There are a great many lights around one of the largest container ports in the country, and what I'm intently looking out for are the red and green lights of the buoys marking the channel to the river Orwell. Indeed, so intently am I aiming for the space between the two that someone is shouting "Have you seen that to your right?", revealing what closely resembles a twenty storey hotel block on its side, motoring on a path that would directly collide with us. I remember the rules of the sea "sail before steam" which somehow doesn't apply in such circumstances. Finally we're in Ipswich moored up.

The ship's mate has also been a git so on washing and hosing the deck I kept losing control of the hose and unfortunately got him rather wet...shame. Bruce, the skipper, left us with the task of cleaning while he went off to see his lady friend. The task he left us was not reasonable; every cupboard and nook and cranny was to be cleaned. This would not have been unreasonable if others using the boat before us had had the same task. However the cobwebs and tins of food that were many years out of date and rusty were a bit of a give-away that we had been the chosen ones to clean away many years worth of dirt out of the boat. We all worked hard for a couple of hours and then Dave decided enough was enough. Bruce was nowhere to be seen. We all downed our tools, leaving most of the contents of the boat on dry land. The captain's mate with his mouth open watched us depart as we got into our cars and headed for home.

As with all these things, unpleasant and dangerous as they are at the time, the overall memory for residents and staff alike is one of achieving something in conditions that were appalling at times. Everyone pulled together, helping each other. The one person who had such a fear is captured in the most wonderful photograph, leaning her chin in her hand gazing out to sea with a most wonderful peaceful and happy smile on her face.

Maggie's Farm

For eleven years we had an annual holiday at Maggie's Farm. Maggie was a mental health social worker who had energy and commitment to her clients and was always prepared to go that 'extra mile'. Each year her small farm would be opened up to staff, day centre clients, Community Support Homes residents, village folk and anybody else who wanted to come along. Wilm, her husband, was the gentle giant for whom nothing was too much trouble. Their generosity and kindness will never be forgotten by so many.

Army mess tents were borrowed, and electricity, toilets and a marquee were all provided. Even a big static caravan for anyone unable to camp for whatever reason was available. Everyone was made welcome. We sang, played games, danced, ate, walked, swam and had a week of fun that so many people enjoyed with their friends and family. Saturday was usually band evening; Wilm's brothers would come and entertain us with their musical talent, alongside other musical friends. Everybody who wanted to join in was included whether it be a song on the mic front of stage or tapping a drum or tambourine on the side. We all loved Maggie's farm holidays; it was one of the highlights of the year!

CHAPTER EIGHT

Mill life was like a tin of Quality Street; people came in many shapes and sizes and various backgrounds (this included the staff!). People were referred to us by social workers or other referring agencies and after our reading their backgrounds and information the individual would be invited to come for a trial visit. It seemed that there was an expectation by the Social Worker and individual that they were turning up for some kind of magic cure and that I had a magic wand. Well obviously in reality life isn't like that, and I didn't have a magic wand. Some effort was expected to be put in on everybody's side. I was certainly going to put in as much effort as I possibly could. Forever the optimist, I believed that people wanted to get better and so I asked what they could offer to the house. Usually people would look flabbergasted, not realising they would have to play an active part in their own recovery. As a consequence we did not accept everyone. What was really important to me was that there was a balance in the house and that whoever came into the house wanted to be there.

On face value residents turmoil would be undetected. S represents how an individual can be perceived to be so together and yet this could not be further from the truth.

"I arrived at the Mill in a blaze of crimson lipstick and cheap nickel chains. This was my adventure into a magical land, the like of which I had never encountered before, and I was embracing it with all my enthusiasm.
Coming as I did from five years spent mostly in the fairly sterile atmosphere of the local psychiatric unit, the Mill with it's sprawling layout, colourful murals and low beamed ceilings, was vibrant. The staff seemed to have arrived straight from Woodstock and my fellow residents ranged from colourful to frankly bizarre; this was definitely the place for me.
The entrance to the Mill was a porch inside which was, amongst other posters and stickers, a sign reading "The Place to Be". Whenever I read it I felt a little less stigmatised and even a little

proud of being part of such an imaginative project.

The hub of the building was neither the staff office nor the lounge, but the kitchen/diner. You were far more likely to find the staff here concocting home made soups of indescribable colours, leading the production line of Christmas wreaths or simply sitting over a cup of tea with visiting CPNs and Social Workers sharing hilarious anecdotes. The Mill was an open and welcoming place whether you were a relative, a social worker or a prospective resident, or even one of the many tradesmen who we relied on to keep the fabric of the building in working order. These workmen in keeping with everything else at the Mill were, shall we say, unconventional. Of particular note were two brothers Wilm and Mitch who were builders, and frequent visitors to the Mill. Wilm was married to Maggie Devine, a hippy Social Worker, who favoured an Indian style of dress and exotic jewellery. Wilm was tall and had long flowing hair and a long beard. His manner was as laid back as his appearance and I never saw him lose his cool or heard him raise his voice. Wilm and Mitch did work hard, where as others were more inclined to drink tea, talk to whoever was about and indulge in trying, usually clumsily, to flirt with Maureen, a blonde, slim and good looking member of staff.

The inhabitants of the Mill were there for a reason however and many of them had almost unbelievably tragic pasts. Whilst all of us were encouraged to leave our pasts and certain related behaviour patterns at the door there were often times when the residents failed to attain the freedom from their life histories that they sought.

In particular many residents struggled with the urge to cut themselves. The motivation for this behaviour was different for each individual, but common threads seem to be a feeling of self loathing and hence the need to punish oneself and the release of pent up emotion. Sometimes there is also the need to have a wound that shows something of the pain going on inside. Whatever the reason, it is also highly addictive behaviour.

I had self harmed as a child and, although I stopped for several years, it became a very entrenched habit when I became ill. When I was struggling to cope with the anger I felt towards myself and others the urge to slash my flesh and see the blood run seemed to satisfy (albeit only temporarily) the need to take some kind of action in response to my inner turmoil. There seemed to be no reason for my agitation and distress and no logic to my actions. I felt like out of control desperate, and violent towards myself. Fortunately I wasn't kicked out and the attitude was 'okay this has happened; now we're going to put it behind us and move on'.

The above story paints a picture of how common sense prevailed over rules and regulations. Dealing with residents was never clearly 'black and white'. Honesty was a big part of community living and generally staff and residents could feel safe in leaving their personal belongings lying around. We resisted locks on doors unless specifically requested by a resident. However, on occasions this trust was broken. What sometimes occurred was a resident 'borrowing' an item without permission, or damaging an item in someone else's room for revenge or theft.

In such situations it is tempting to create rules to prevent a re-occurrence. However, we felt strongly that rules are not the answer and in fact can create additional pressures on residents and staff.

When something did happen the issue would be confronted usually by calling the whole house together, explaining what the problem was and how it could be resolved. We would look at ways for people to return things without humiliation and understand the implications of their actions by being more in touch with their conscience.

Before an individual was accepted into the house we would encourage them to visit regularly, but preferably stay for a few days, so that they could be assessed by us and the views of the residents considered. Sometimes residents felt quite strongly that somebody shouldn't move in. However, people came with a variety of issues, some very complex, and in general the residents were very tolerant of this. As far as possible we would avoid taking residents who mirrored similar behaviours; for instance, having two young men both with severe schizophrenia or challenging behaviour. It was important to be aware of group dynamics and to maintain a balance of individual's difficulties for staff and for residents living within the group. We were also very aware of collusion between residents, especially individuals with alcohol or drug dependency. We strove towards a 'family feeling' and therefore considered a mixed age range to be the most beneficial way for residents to recuperate from mental illness. Our philosophy was based on the concept of an extended family unit.

We felt the bigger the mix the better it was; also we tried to avoid having too many residents of the same age group. For instance, too many youngsters together would be like living in a youth club, which could get a bit rowdy and out of hand. However, it was good if some of the older residents could impart their wisdom to the younger ones, and they in turn energise them. We would encourage them to laugh and think and care about somebody else apart from themselves. A lot of thought was put into creating good group dynamics. Any new resident coming into the house would affect the balance of the house and the 'pecking order' just like any family. Sometimes a prospective resident would be full of self doubt and totally lacking in confidence, believing that they could never change. However, my 'gut instinct' and optimism that people can change would be sufficient to persuade them to trust us and join the group if only for the trial period.

Certainly some of the people who lived in our house needed intensive input, whilst others needed gentle support and guidance on their day to day living basis, and there was always somebody around providing good 'role modelling.' I recall a lad who I will call Paul, brought to us by his Social Worker, and who lived in one of the little market towns nearby. He sat completely mute in our meeting and when people behaved like this I tried to include them but not in an obvious way. So as I talked to the Social Worker I'd be looking for the lad's responses, his eyes brightening up or engaging slightly towards me, but I would still chatter on. I would laugh a bit, to make him relax. I would ask him a question and he would grunt and answer here and there. Having read his notes before he came, I knew that he had a bicycle, and I instantly identified a way forward into this lad's head. I would always try to discover what an individual's interests were and aim to engage with them with this in mind.

So I said to this lad "Oh, do you still ride a bike? I heard that you had your own bicycle and that you used to bike into town sometimes," and he immediately replied that he did. Then I asked if he had any skills he could bring to the house. Could he cook? "No." Could he clean? "No." Could he look after himself? "No." Everything was 'No'. So I told him I had a bike in the garage that had two punctured tyres and asked him if he could mend them because I had not got the foggiest idea of how to do it. It was like somebody had just switched the light on. He smiled and indicated he would be delighted to fix my punctures. So it is just a question of finding a way in and breaking the ice. I would challenge a young person by reminding them that they initially said they could not do anything and then pointing out to them that in fact they could.

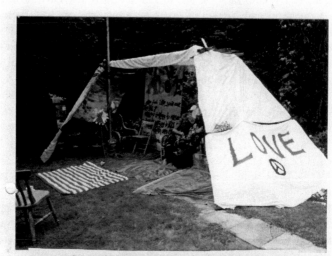

Peter and Sal enjoying 'Hippy Day' in the Mill garden

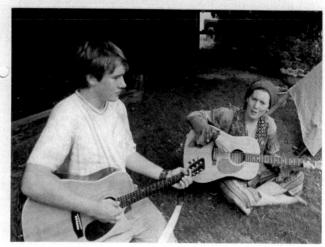

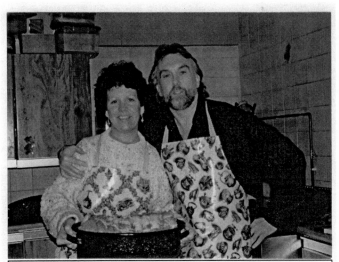

(*above*) Helen and Dave in The Mill kitchen – the centre of daily activity

(*below*) Blockfest at the Devine's Farm – such good times!

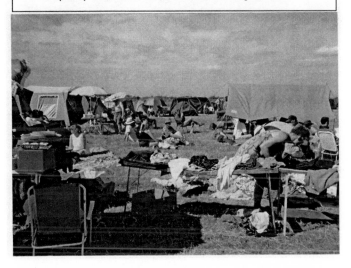

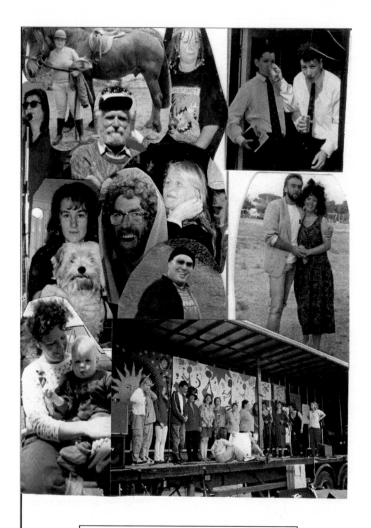

Too many folk to mention but great memories

CHAPTER NINE

For the first time in my life I had such a hunger for information and a desire to help out in the mental health field that I couldn't find out enough about it all to satisfy myself. I found text books difficult to engage with because I am dyslexic and believe this encouraged me to think creatively about how I interacted with residents. I think that my upbringing gave me a 'toolbox' of skills to make sense of all the different individuals who would come in. I suppose my 'mother nature' instinct and my life experiences took the place of theoretical learning. A lot of this experience came from working with young offenders, young people, voluntary involvement with toddler groups and the elderly.

I attended a counselling course which was intensive formal learning and included residential weekends. The majority of students on the course were professionals working in the mental health field who had quite impressive backgrounds. I had absolutely no knowledge about anything to do with social care and I felt about an inch tall on my first day on the course, considering that these people had seen it, done it, knew it. I was on this course for a year. It seemed most of the group had experienced some traumatic events in their own lives. However, I did not feel this applied to me and almost felt obliged to make up a history to fit in. I was feeling so uncomfortable with the thought of sitting in on one particular group leader's session that I made up a story, saying I felt that there would be potential transference from my mother if I did. I felt there were far more interesting group leaders to be with than her, and already I was trying to manipulate the groups and the systems to where I wanted to be. Everyone else in the group had a wealth of experience and were professionals in the field of mental health from whom I learnt a lot. Overall it was a great learning experience for me and by the time I left I really did feel like my self esteem and confidence were in a much better place. I certainly lost any sense of feeling inferior and discovered that I had more knowledge than I had given myself credit for. I believe, despite our backgrounds, we all have fantasies and skeletons in our cupboards which can affect our confidence, self worth and judgement, leading us to believe that others know best.

.

It seemed to me that common sense brought about the same results with less effort via simple straightforward communication. On one occasion we were set up in small groups with Lego and straws to make a 'creation' whilst being observed by the group leaders. Their task was to ascertain our behaviour within the group setting to determine what role we chose for ourselves within the group, such as communication skills, taking the lead or being led etc. Attending this course whetted my appetite for knowledge and encouraged me to gain relevant qualifications. I also dipped my toe briefly into Psychotherapy and NLP (Neuro Linguistic Programming), both of which added to my 'tool box'. I always feel that care should be taken when dipping into a little bit of theory here and there. I was amazed by some of the theories and convoluted explanations for human behaviour that were second nature to me. It is dangerous to play around with people's minds and easy to fall into the trap of thinking, after attending a training course, that we can apply our new found knowledge and successfully solve people's problems. I recall a conversation with Dr Morgan, a Consultant Psychiatrist, who I deeply respected, and he stated that he believed extreme caution was needed concerning the intervention of newly qualified 'Counsellors' keen to apply their new found skills too quickly and running the risk of leaving their clients vulnerable. I have always felt that it is too easy to expose levels of distress in an individual, by delving deeply into their feelings, and not respecting that time is needed to assist them in dealing with what they uncover. I strongly believe that people need to be able to 'put the lid back on' the potential 'can of worms'.

To illustrate the complexities of mental illness and the effects it has on an individual, especially schizophrenia, I will give you a flavour of just how terrifying it can be by relating the stories of two people. I have altered some facts to protect anonymity.

R was 23 when his mother died. He was estranged from his

brother who lived away. After the death of his mother, R's mental health deteriorated and he developed schizophrenia. Unfortunately this was not diagnosed, which meant he did not receive any support. He lived on his own on a property of approximately a quarter of an acre. R became convinced that evil spirits had come to their home and killed his mother and so he had to protect himself. He became obsessed by this, and he began barricading himself into his garden and house by gathering every piece of wood he could find and nailing them together. Each day he did this and it began to look like an obscure piece of art. It took him some time to achieve a total barricade of the grounds. When the whole perimeter was securely enclosed he painted signs and symbols which would keep the evil spirits out. He then began on the house, boarding up and painting each and every window with his signs and symbols, putting the house into complete darkness. Eventually he did not feel safe in his small bedroom and moved into a tiny cellar under the stairs, which I think at one time had been an inspection pit for repairing cars. I'm not sure how long he remained there but fortunately a neighbour rang the police to report they could hear a dog whimpering. When the police arrived they found two dead dogs and an emaciated mongrel lying next to the hatch of the inspection pit. They lifted the hatch and found R huddled in a corner hiding his face with one hand and holding a wooden spear in the other. He was emaciated, filthy, paranoid, frightened and totally detached from reality. Can you imagine the injustice of the effects of this illness on someone who was previously successful in his own business, intelligent, was leading what appeared to be a normal life and had plans for his future? The above illustrates how the onset of mental illness can creep into somebody's life and take over.

The second individual, who I will call Sue, came from a good supportive family and excelled at school academically and in sport. In her late teens she indulged in recreational drugs to excess and this sparked off schizophrenia which was also a hereditary factor within the family. I have known her for twenty years and I think she is the most tortured soul I have met. She would constantly hear voices, some happy ones and some unhappy destructive ones. These voices would take on a character of their own and she believed they were real people talking to her in her head. One voice in particular identified itself as a well known figure who Sue believed instructed her to carry out many bizarre rituals that resulted in physical damage to her body. It also told her the world was going to end and Sue was the 'chosen one' and important in preventing this. After numerous bizarre events that involved the police and Social Workers she was eventually sectioned under the Mental Health Act and taken to a secure hospital. She escaped, stole a credit card from a mutual friend and, in nothing else than the clothes she wore when she escaped, travelled on a one way ticket to find the character who had issued her with his instructions. Given that the voices in her head were not real it is not surprising that she was unable to find him. She then panicked and rang me at the Mill. I told her she needed to return as soon as possible! She did so using the same credit card but I had ensured this person knew what was happening. I informed the relevant services and she was escorted from the airport back to the Secure Unit.

Sometimes I would challenge her voices, saying to her 'Have they ever been right? Why should they be right now then?' To do this I found I had to get on her level, and if she was screaming and shouting I would have to adopt a number of different approaches based on my gut feelings to get her attention! Sometimes she would explode with anger and frustration and at others she would calm down and listen.

Not long after returning from this trip half way round the world, and placed back into the secure hospital, she escaped again, only this time she stole a vehicle and arrived at the Mill with her head shaved "to keep the devils away". She looked absolutely mad. I need to explain here that when dealing with extreme bizarre behaviour like this, rational thought sometimes gets lost by the worker involved! I believe my thinking was also affected by the fact that I was heavily pregnant at the time and the birth was imminent! Anyway, I felt I wanted to protect Sue from being arrested, knowing how distressed she would become, and decided I had to get the vehicle away from the Mill which I did by moving it to a street in the village. Also I wanted to get her away from the Mill for the sake of the residents and my family. I got her into my car to take her to a family member as a temporary measure, knowing she would not willingly go back to the hospital unit. As soon as we set off she scrambled down into the passenger foot well and kept rubbing her hands up and down my legs! I asked her whatever did she think she was doing and to stop at once, which she did! She then agreed to sit in the passenger seat. I tried different people with whom she could stay but none were at home. At one point we passed a police car in a lay by which caused Sue to dive back down into the foot well, ranting and terrified. In the end I managed to persuade her to go to another friend she had thought of who fortunately took her in. I arrived back at the Mill and was confronted by Dave who was beside himself with worry which he expressed through extreme anger! That was one of only two occasions when I have seen him "lose it"!

There are many different routes as to why we have been involved with the rehabilitation and care of different individuals. The next story is told by a woman who has had a traumatic past, which led her to our care.

This is Brenda's life's journey and I have left it as close as possible to her own account.

Brenda

By the time I was six my brother and I had been moved into care because of our abusive home life. We had lived in a family which was based on poverty, fear, alcohol abuse and violence. Mum was soon to jump out of the frying pan and into the fire. Mum left Dad and was soon remarried. I now had a step-dad and a new baby brother who would join us on the 'at risk' register. At a month old my step-brother was found with a cigarette burn on him and it was then that we were put into care.

After four years of being the youngest kids at the Orchards Home in Wisbech we returned home. Sadly it didn't work out for me. I was made to sleep in a 'bedroom' under the stairs and was regularly beaten with a mop or broom. Mum would leave me in the dark to punish me, meaning that I couldn't read my 'Bunty' books. She would shout "Turn the fucking light off". I was scared.

When I was twelve I drank a bottle of disinfectant and had to go to hospital to have my stomach pumped. I was soon returned to care after this.

I went to a school for children with special needs as my behaviour was disruptive and unmanageable. After this I was transferred to a live-in school where I did well and enjoyed sport and art. I worked hard and got on well with the group although at times my anger would get the better of me and I would be restrained.

At thirteen I needed twelve stitches after self-harming. I think I did it because I felt tortured. I missed my Mum yet I was so scared of her.

At sixteen I moved to a psychiatric unit for children called 'Douglas House. They worked towards me and Mum becoming reunited but I couldn't cope even though I really wanted to.

I moved into a shared house with three other girls. My move lasted seven months. It was chaos. The other girls beat me up and called me a 'psycho'. The house share came to an end when they pushed my head through a window and I was admitted to hospital. I moved to another kids resource called the 'Old Rectory' for two weeks while I waited for a bed at Mill House. I overdosed and cut my arms here as I felt so alone.

I moved into the Mill with the lovely Helen and Dave. I enjoyed the Mill – we went swimming, on trips to the beach and to Sandringham. We did carol singing. That was fun. I couldn't sing, well most of us couldn't, but we got the money. We went to Derbyshire on holiday where I rode a horse, went rock climbing and abseiled. I felt confident and part of a family and I felt like I belonged.

I was soon to meet Eddie at the Mill and we became soul mates and inseparable. We both loved the Mill - eating round the table, living in a family atmosphere, feeling wanted, loved and needed. We felt independent and yet we felt like we belonged.

After eighteen months I had learnt to cook, pay bills and manage our money. We felt more confident and emotionally stronger. We moved out of the Mill and into a place together. In the early days we sometimes struggled. I would turn to drink and cut myself. Some people can't help self harming no matter what anyone else says.

Let me tell you about Eddie. Eddie and his two sisters suffered from schizophrenia. Elaine jumped off the Arndale Centre in Leeds and Viv died from a massive drugs overdose. His dad was dead and his mum hadn't spoken to him since he was a teenager. At fourteen Eddie moved in with a school caretaker who was sexually abusing him. This damaged our physical relationship as he always felt dirty.

His life became chaotic as a result of the illness which led to deviant behaviour that led to custody. He also took drugs to stop the voices. Unfortunately the drugs he took only made matters worse. He used to sit and talk to the wall. He liked riding his motorbike and his deluded ideas and voices in his head would tell him he wouldn't crash and fortunately he didn't. After being deemed a danger to himself and others he was placed in a secure unit for six years. He believed that a priest in the secure unit had made Jesus come into his life which haunted him and made him very distressed and paranoid. He spent most of the time in a state of paranoia believing people were talking about him which made him incredibly anxious.

Many types and doses of medication were tried because he was medication resistant due to the intensity of his illness. He moved out of the secure unit into the Fermoy psychiatric hospital waiting for a place in the Mill. He had an excellent social worker, Maggie, who we both thought was brilliant.

Eddie and I met at the Mill. I married him two months before my twentieth birthday, and we were married fifteen years. Every day was a roller coaster because of his paranoia and each day there would be a need for reassurance. We were soul mates, we just clicked, and we spent twenty four hours a day together. We loved each other very much and I still miss his smile. I'll always call him an idiot for committing suicide. He dived in front of a car. I don't know how desperate he must have been to do it.

Earlier that same evening he'd tried to electrocute himself. I spoke to him on the phone and begged him not to do anything silly which he promised he wouldn't. He swore on his love to me, and usually when we did that to each other, we'd stick to it. Within minutes of leaving the phone box he had thrown himself under the wheels of an oncoming car. In his desperate and anxious state he had failed to put anything on his feet.

Prior to all of this I had begged the services to help him and keep him safe. My words to them fell on deaf ears and the consequences have been devastating.

At the inquest I met the people who ran over him. They were gutted, they were in a mess, so I thought I've got to make them feel better because I can't leave it like this. I reassured them it wasn't their fault, not to blame themselves. They said thank you very much and cried their eyes out.

Can you imagine what it must feel like to lose your 20year old son in a road traffic accident? An ordinary hard-working couple called Gary and June not only had the relentless grief of losing their son, they then had the trauma of running over Eddie who had a history of psychiatric problems. Gary tells their story;

"We were going to visit my Mum. It was about 4.30 on a sunny afternoon. We were driving down North Lynn when a red car in front of us swerved across the road. We saw a man standing on the curb of the pavement and presumed he had been dropped off by the red car. We were travelling very slowly over the speed bumps and I said "Look at him, he is off his face". I presumed

he was very pissed or high on drugs, he looked terrible. As we got closer he peered into the car, his enormous eyes and face willing us to look at him. When the car was almost parallel with him he dived like a footballer. The car went over him in what felt like slow motion. We were both stunned into silence. June opened her passenger door and there next to her were Eddie's battered and bruised ankles and feet. I shouted at her to get in the drivers seat and leapt out of the car in order to lift it off Eddie while she put the car in reverse which in fact she didn't need to do. One eye witness ran over to help and between us we lifted the car off Eddie. I had already called to another householder to call the police and ambulance as our normally very reliable mobile phones were without a signal. I asked the witness to stay with Eddie until the services arrived. I needed to stand beside the open door to comfort June who was now in a hideous state of shock, as was I. The ambulance and police seemed to take forever to arrive although it was probably only minutes."

They had to strap Eddie to the stretcher because he kept fighting to get up, he had been held down on the road by the chap who helped lift the car off him. The police questioned Gary and June while waiting for a variety of road accident specialists to arrive including a team from Swaffham who fine tooth combed the car to ensure there were no faults with the Renault Scenic they were driving. June's physical state worried Gary and eventually after several hours and him having to get very firm with the police they left to go home. Gary remained at the accident spot until 9.30 pm, more than five hours. Confused and exhausted, the police told him he could go. He doesn't know how he drove the car home that night and looks back in wonderment at the police allowing him to drive as he clearly wasn't safe. On arriving home he and June started to unravel what had happened to them. A resurrection of feelings had flooded back to them on the loss of their precious son. How they had cordoned off the road with tape at each end. How the lights of the investigating team from Swaffham with their powerful lighting had lit the road up.

At 11 o'clock the phone rang to say Eddie was dead. The news hit them like a ton of bricks. The call from the police was brief and to the point. Gary said to June "I've killed someone's son, husband or father. I've lost my own son and now I've killed somebody else's".

Their distress and grief consumed them throughout the night and the next day. They felt to blame. The following afternoon at about 4.30 the police came to the door. "We hadn't had any contact until this point apart from the call to tell us he was dead. We were separated into different rooms to give our statements" June said. "We were made to feel like criminals".

A difficult journey was to follow and Gary and June appreciate that had they not lost their son maybe their grief wouldn't have been so hard. Sleep became a thing of the past, a couple of hours here and there. Flashbacks were a daily reminder of the day in question. Eddie's screaming and the smell of his burning flesh beneath the car. The feelings of panic to lift the car off him and the strength needed that came from within. Eddie's blood that poured between Gary's legs and feet as he looked under and lifted the car. Kids that had gathered at the scene shouting "Have you killed him, is he dead?". Gary can still hear their voices, see Eddie's face, his eyes, his burns, the scene, the inquest. Gary couldn't face work, he couldn't cope with anyone asking how he was or asking for details of the crash. He couldn't face going out of the house. Gary says "I have suffered worse when my son died but this stopped me in my tracks. I left my job; I was depressed and unable to function. A woman came from victim support for a few weeks but I'm sorry to say she was of no help. She lacked experience and talked about her own past experiences and problems. I don't think she could have been trained. We sold the car and I found a new job where I could be anonymous. My friends used to say 'Gary, go to a solicitor, get some compensation' – they didn't understand that compensation was the last thing on my mind. I didn't want to be greedy and I wasn't interested. I had no self preservation or motivation. Me and June just got through each day. We still do. We went to our doctor who could offer no help apart from a referral to psychiatric services".

Gary felt he was too frightened to go, he felt that he would be kept in hospital and trapped in a system once they knew how unstable and fragile he was. June was no longer able to travel in the passenger seat of their new car. Both of them suffer anxiety when driving or being a passenger and they watch with intensity in case anyone falls or jumps off the curb. In the last few years they have moved house five times. Gary says "June and I can't keep running"; the trouble is, the pain continues to run with them.

Gary feels angry with Eddie. June can now feel for Eddie knowing he was so unwell. They both feel let down by the system and angry with it! They don't know who was responsible for Eddie's care and they feel he should have been in hospital. The police explained to them that he had tried to electrocute himself and stab himself prior to the incident. At the time they didn't digest this information and didn't want to. They could only think that they had killed someone, leaving them both in a very deep black hole. Gary says "I expect it's f***ing money that stopped him getting the help he needed. Now we are left to suffer the consequences of his lack of care. The system failed to look after us and Eddie. People who have the power to make the decisions to keep people safe should use them because they wouldn't want to carry the memories and mental scars that me and June now have to live with."

The onset of mental illness may seem to come as a result of trauma or a period of stressful life events. For some people there seems to be no rhyme or reason. However, often, in my experience, there are tell tale signs much earlier on in an individual's life that have been overlooked or deemed not particularly relevant. As below it can often be a case of drowning not waving.

Descent into Chaos:

Told by an ex Mill resident:

Looking back, I can see that there were signs of emotional instability fairly early on in childhood but it wasn't until my late twenties that a crisis arose in my life and was to lead me into nightmare scenarios for over a decade.

At the age of twenty seven I had ascended from temporary gift vouchers girl to Sales Manager of a large department store. Although I had been a success story as a supervisor I hated my new job and for a year my failures grew with my stress levels. Each night I would go home screaming for a way out. I was unable to sleep and often started work at 1am. All I wanted to talk about to anyone was my desperation. I couldn't afford to resign, had no insight into the mental breakdown I was heading for and just waited in hope of a heart attack. Finally an appalling area inspection led to disciplinary action. Eventually I ceased to function at all, cried incessantly and became incapable of performing the simplest tasks. I had no choice but to go to my GP.

I was fortunate that my doctor took time to listen and ask pertinent questions and made follow up appointments for me. Anti-depressants however failed to elevate my mood and as a consequence of admitting suicidal feelings I was admitted to the local psychiatric hospital for the first of many stays. Over the next five years I was a prisoner to low moods when I would harm myself with anything I could get hold of. I learned to steal light bulbs from other people's bed cubicles and wrap them in a towel when smashing them to deaden the sound before I cut myself with the glass. On going into town I would purchase razor blades for more serious damage. The impact on my family was devastating as they watched their daughter / sister fall into a horrific abyss that they couldn't begin to understand or control.

There was, however, another side to my experience which

although sometimes enjoyable could be equally destructive. At times my mood would soar, I would have the energy to stay awake long after everyone else had been worn out by my non-stop dialogue (no, make that monologue). Money meant nothing to me. I would buy extravagant gifts and emerge laden from expensive art galleries - all on the plastic, of course. I truly believed that I was fabulously rich and that lavish living was mine. Changes of routine were fatal and I have had to leave holidays after the last one led to delusions of my role as prophet to the nation and planned certain inappropriate action outside no. 10. Before you conclude that this all sounds more like great fun than illness, let me say a word or two. People do get tired of you, being black listed isn't much fun and even delusions of grandeur get frustrating. On top of this is the feeling that things are getting faster and faster and that you're not quite in control. Then comes the drop, and boy is it a long way down and even though you know they're right you want to punch the person who tells you a good walk and fresh air will make you feel so much better.

I wish I could give you a 'cure for all' recipe for complete recovery but bi-polar is a different experience for different people and what works for one person won't for someone else. I can however share what has and hasn't worked for me. Bad as being in hospital was, it was better than being on my own at my lowest points. I was lucky that in that at least some of the staff seemed to care and exercised some creativity in their approach towards me. It was the place I needed to be when I needed to be protected from myself. In time, however, I needed longer term solutions to my need for supported accommodation and care (incidentally I am convinced that the lack of this is responsible for much cost and human suffering) and I sought out a therapeutic community. Based on principles of respect and responsibility I found what for me was the foundation of rebuilding self-esteem. Every achievement was noted and supported and when you've probably lost the ability to value yourself that is enormously helpful. Equally helpful was a no nonsense approach and the ability for someone to put the brakes on and introduce a bit of reality. Medication can be helpful for some, and new options are available. A good relationship with your G.P. and/or CPN and Psychiatrist is a great help, especially if you live independently. Much as I know it can be the last thing on earth you want to do, try and get exercise and engage with your local community. A little bit of reading around food and drink can give some helpful insights into self help, and if you can get some recommended reading around the issues you have to deal with that's good, although don't label yourself too much. Finally, although obviously not conclusively, don't think that you will always feel the same.

Undoubtedly the Mill saved my life and allowed me to have a future.

We had many social work students on placement with us at the Mill. Without exception their feedback was always positive. Although they recognised that the formula in operation at the Mill without question worked they were at a loss as to how to present this in an academic format. This was not the case for some of the student psychiatric nurses on placement who found that the lack of black and white thinking was an uncomfortable working environment. Some could not comprehend the ethos behind the Mill's philosophy and therefore were totally lacking in respect towards both staff and residents. I wouldn't dream of tarring them all with the same brush as there were many outstanding exceptions, to whom I will remain always grateful for their special input, commitment and hard work. Perhaps we should be less than surprised at the difficulty some had in comprehending the day to day living and workings of the Mill.

CHAPTER TEN

What follows is a loose snapshot of our day to day living reminisced by Catherine and myself. Catherine is an ex resident who is now a good friend.

A week in the life of The Mill:

Monday

Monday morning always begins with the staff bundling into the Mill after a weekend of skeleton staff and peace (usually!) This almost certainly symbolizes the start of a manic week.

Dave is greeted by Terry as normal, who announces "f**k off back up the bungalow Dave, we don't need you here" at the top of his voice.

"And good morning to you Terry" Dave replies.

Mondays are notoriously busy. There is always a full house and a lot of noise. To begin, staff gather around the kitchen table for a general chit chat which seems to ease them into the working day. Eventually the residents follow suit and join staff at the table. Occasionally, in depth discussions about current affairs take place, with everybody around the table putting their point across. And there is always tons of laughter. This simple exercise seems to enforce the union of staff and residents being on an equal footing.

As residents quickly appear, some are still in yesterday's (or dare we say last week's) clothes. Dry food, cigarette burns and great splashes of coffee the complete norm on one's attire. Dishevelled hair inclining to one side and socks half on and half off, almost tripping oneself up with each sleepy footstep. Other residents are smartly dressed in appropriate casual clothing. The odd resident may need encouragement to put on a bra, or change from something that looks more respectable for a Monday than a short skirt and high heels. "We are not going clubbing this morning, you will catch your death, go and get something warm on." (Staff and residents did go clubbing quite regularly, we loved a good boogie and a night out) . Not only did residents dress inappropriately, on more than one occasion students needed guidance as to appropriate dress. I recall one nursing student turning up on her first day's work in six inch heels looking sexy and ready for a pole dancing session. In fact she told me that at weekends she was a pole dancer to earn extra cash whilst on her course. Although this was much approved of by some of the male staff and residents we strived to have some decorum. In my own mind I thought "How on earth is she going to muck out rooms, mop floors or help in the garden". After the first day when she had been busy pitching in with all the practical duties she was absolutely crippled and dishevelled by the time she finished her shift. She did become an asset to the house. Flat shoes, casual trousers and non revealing tops became her normal dress after her first day! I often used to have to whisper in people's ears about appropriate dress.

Monday is house shop day. A duty not to be wished on even the most efficient person. The first task is to round the 'shoppers' up. This is very difficult in itself, taking forever at times. It is quite normal to see staff running up and down the stairs trying to round everybody up, and get them in the same place at the same time. Encouraging people from the depths of their duvets who have been up all night and only asleep for 20 minutes.

Residents seem to have all sorts of problems with the shopping chores, with Sandra announcing that she cannot possibly help with the shopping because she is wearing an itchy bra and Marie struggling with her personal shopping list because at the minute she can only eat red food! Requests for the shopping list was a thoughtful task for everyone living at the Mill. Each week a request list would be put on the kitchen whiteboard. If you wanted Marmite or gooseberry jam etc. etc. it would be the individual's responsibility to put it on the whiteboard. As the week progressed the list would grow in size and then we had to extract the ingredients needed for the menus that had been agreed at the house meeting. We then had the instant 'fancies' from those gathered around the kitchen table whilst putting the list together. Depending on how hungry people felt the list could become very large – people always seem to want an enormous shop when they are hungry. After rounding everybody up and making it as far as the check-out the tricky job of unloading and packing three or more overflowing trolleys (yes, quite literally) commences. Twenty or so loaves of bread are purchased along with kilos and kilos of potatoes and every other item multiplied by an astounding amount to feed the hungry Millers for a week. Shopping wasn't always a smooth operation and the following accounts will give a flavour of some of the trials and tribulations. Self catering was done by residents living in the attached cottage and bed-sits within the main house. They had responsibility for their own menus and shopping list. There were criteria to adhere to which meant a healthy diet, not Coke, chocolate or beer etc. However, there was often someone out on a scam producing receipts with a footprint on that had been collected off the floor and clearly not their receipt. Others would attempt to buy fags or pocket a bit of the money. Then there was Karen who would pop off to Marks and Spencer, pay on her store card, buy too much lavish food that she couldn't afford and have it delivered to the Mill, using the budget cash to suck on posh cigars whilst waiting for her booty to arrive! (she was always a little grandiose!). So, after purchasing half the supermarket and making it home without losing anybody (ah, not so every week!) the shopping is put away by any unsuspecting person available. This task is detested by most residents who would much rather be hiding in a corner with a cigarette and a coffee. Helen always seems to have the powers of persuasion for such events, cheerily telling the 'lazy lumps' to put their cigarette down for a minute and help with the shopping. "We are all going to enjoy eating this food" she would say. "Come on, come on", and if the wheel barrow was handy, with a smile she would load the shopping in and wheel it round the back of the house to the store cupboard.

The weekly house meeting is also held on a Monday in the evening. Residents are retrieved from obscure hiding places around the Mill and brought together in the living room to air any difficulties. Residents had mixed feelings about house meetings. They could be exciting as we discussed trips and activities for the following week and longer term events or outings. I would chair the meeting, always making sure that all points of view were listened to. At times opinions could clash and become heated, but reassurance was given that the need to respect everybody's views was important. We didn't have to agree, and sometimes we would challenge a person's thinking. But the meetings were all for freedom of speech. Monday meetings were compulsory to attend as the forum and information affected all of our community. Some people said very little, but it was always a good feeling for me when an unexpected resident would speak up. The bond in the house with each other became very strong and at times I think this helped people's recovery. Without the feeling of safety moving forward seems impossible. Dave was always available with his very calm persona. He was like the wise owl and would speak with pertinence when needed. His views were always respected and listened to. Dave, residents and staff I'm sure thought I had too much to say, but that was me. So, we all come together in the lounge and find a place to sit and it is at this point every week, while everyone is seated, that Andrew decides to go for a stroll up and down the living room and kitchen, the door slamming behind him each time he crosses the rooms. A tall fellow, with his hands behind his back, he continuously roams, almost stepping on toes and obviously deciding that his evening walk beats sitting in a room full of moaning people, laughing people, anxious and thoughtful people. Helen always managed to make those meetings thought provoking!

First thing on the meeting agenda is deciding on the menu for the following week. All residents are encouraged to request a meal that they would like but there was a catch however, whatever you choose you must help prepare for twenty plus people. Meal ideas seem to change with the different personalities of changing residents. Some decide that perhaps haggis or tripe may be good things to try, or Mexican or Italian nights, while others think that your bog standard Shepherd's Pie will do just fine. Arduous topics are often brought up such as stealing, and there is obviously an apt way of dealing with such issues. Personal differences and tricky situations are dealt with at house meetings and this is a time for staff and residents to voice their concerns. There is an agenda that is followed, where residents and staff are able to bring up any difficulties. It is kept on the kitchen door at all times and people add things as they so wish. The thing brought up almost weekly was used cups being left about – the absolute bain of Mill life. For some reason those damn cups never made it to a bowl full of soapy water very often (unless repeatedly reminded by staff)!

At the end of the house meeting an enormous basket of washing (who knows if it was all clean or not) was emptied onto the floor so people could retrieve their long forgotten items; items which had occasionally been left hanging about for quite some time. "Whose knickers are these"? was a familiar question. With over twenty residents such items were occasionally 'shared', and so the knickers never quite belonged to anybody, or, more interestingly, everyone!

We had a lot of laughs and a lot of moans. We tried really hard to include all residents in the meeting, although this proved difficult at times with the odd resident wandering in and out of the room, unable to sit and concentrate for any length of time. We would gently encourage those with difficulties around talking within groups to try and build their self-confidence; everybody has a right to be heard and respected. It was not only important to build the self-esteem of residents; staff would sometimes need to build up their confidence in order to handle a large group, where there maybe conflict, lethargy, interruptions from those who always had plenty to say and inclusion of those with anxiety, depression and feelings of emptiness which kept them hidden in one of the corners. It was a real skill to manage successfully.

Tuesday

Residents are asked to do a daily chore such as cleaning the kitchen floor or hoovering the hallway. It has ALWAYS been hard and probably ALWAYS will be. While some residents are eager, such as Mrs S who made a great effort to rise really early to clean the kitchen floor before the rest of the house woke so that at least there was half a chance that it would keep clean for a while! The kitchen floor was a never ending job. Some residents had a knack of making a cup of coffee in the kitchen and leaving a great trail of it as they walked through to the living room. Hence a constant stream of sticky coffee on the floors and an extraordinary mess around the kettle which would never be clean for long even if you followed everybody around with a cloth! This really got to a sweet older lady who would spend the whole day muttering under her breath about the 'lazy, bloody b*****ds' as she attempted to clean the area as best as she could while at the same time pocketing biscuits and hiding mixtures of cake and pickle under her dress for a snack later on!

It would be fair to say that a lot of the residents just weren't keen on the daily house jobs and would try to get out of it if at all possible. Staying in bed was a favourite avoidance technique used by many, going out early another or a simple 'f*ck off' another!
Staff member Angie was very particular about corners, much to the agony of the residents. She would often be seen pulling out furniture and 'showing' the unenthusiastic bunch the art of deep cleaning. Other residents were more willing however; for example, after being asked to hoover, one chap could be seen putting all his might into the chore - the only snag being that he was hoovering the back patio!

An ongoing task on a Tuesday was the vegetable shopping. This was fairly plain sailing on the whole. Helen would go to the market at the end of the day and was renowned for buying bargain boxes of reduced priced fruit and veg. This was a great idea in itself, except for the fact that the poor staff member that evening, usually Chris, would have to chop the vegetables, blanch them and separate them into freezer bags to be used at a later date. It wasn't just a little box however, it was enormous, and after six hours it would probably be done. The funniest thing was that Helen would always start the conversation with "If you could just…." Helen and Dave would always insist that healthy food is good food; healthy meals are a good start to a healthy mind. Nothing was wasted; there was a place for everything, whether it was made into endless pans of multicoloured soup, or great batches of hotpot or casserole! This brings us on to teatime. Usually a good time for the ever hungry Millers! The poor chefs for the evening wouldn't always have such a great time, however! They would at times need to cater for five special diets as well as preparing the main dish. Vegetarian, low potassium, low fat, diabetic and chicken-only were all catered for. An extremely hard task to attempt, especially as people not on any form of special diet would decide that that evening they didn't fancy their prepared meal and would quite like to try one of the others. Fine, as it stands; everybody was encouraged to make choices and what have you, but there was only a certain amount of the 'special' meals. One lady, for instance, would stand over the chefs and inspect what was on offer. She would turn her nose up at her requested meal, stating "hmm, I want that over there" and if refused would storm off in an absolute temper shouting "I won't eat any f***ing grub at all then".

At mealtimes another chap would have to be coaxed into eating, as from the moment he woke up in the morning he would state loudly and constantly "I don't want any tea tonight, I'm not hungry". He could usually be encouraged to eat something, after shouting "You fat gannets" at the seated diners if he was a bit high!

Andrew would be very interested in the cooking process, often enquiring about the food being cooked etc., but when it came to teatime he would almost certainly refuse the meal, but would occasionally settle for a bowl of bananas and custard! It was a real family occasion, eating together. A rather elderly lady would usually be seated in the middle of our large farmhouse table. She was a well spoken lady of royal ancestry and would take small bites at a time. However, more often than not she would choke on a piece of meat for instance, and would begin coughing ferociously before a desperate tap on the back would release the food from her throat which would consequently fly across the table!

After a usually very tasty meal, the washing up was the next task on the agenda. Over the years numerous techniques have been used to make sure everybody pulled their weight, seeing as it is the least popular job among the Millers. Rotas were put together, requesting different named residents washed up, dried up and washed the floor on a certain day. When this didn't work, Millers were asked to wash their own knife, fork and plate and one pan each. Elaborate excuses were made almost nightly. One lady would suddenly be struck with tremendous pain and, patting her leg, would say "It's an old tennis injury dear. I don't think I can wash up, it's too painful". This certain 'injury' had occurred literally fifty or so years before! Staff were always left with more than their fair share. The energy to keep it all 'rolling' would wane and the staff would quietly finish the task.

Wednesday

Wednesday - Mill House choir practice. Chrissy would come and teach choir members a number of songs from around the world. You could not always guarantee that members would be very enthusiastic about practice, the novelty having worn off very quickly for some. This, however, was not an acceptable excuse as at the Mill 'commitment' was a 'buzz word'. Once you had agreed to do something you did it come hell or high water. Positive peer pressure was always at hand. Part of the philosophy at the Mill was to keep the mind occupied, the body active and the spirit uplifted. This was seen as preparation for a time when self motivation was essential for future success in the community.

So, there they are, the members of the Mill Choir, those who at first resisted, now enjoying themselves thoroughly (another reason why commitment is so treasured). The tangle of voices putting heart and soul into each song, a grin from ear to ear. One lady comes to mind who would engage in the experience with enthusiasm, balancing her glasses on the end of her nose, whilst heavily laden with an assortment of jewellery. She demanded the limelight and could often be seen swiping the microphone from a more timid participant!

Unfortunately enthusiasm didn't stretch to the reluctant listeners in the other room having a 'quiet' fag and coffee! They would be put through 'extreme torture' because of the melodies coming from the conservatory. "It's a heap of sh*t, none of you can sing" one man announced when asked what he thought of our choir. The singers didn't always stay in the conservatory, much to the others' annoyance. There was one song "Zum gali gali gali, zum gali gali, zum gali gali gali zum" which would be repeated in a round while at the same time walking all around the Mill, hands on the shoulders in front of you and a hearty kick to the side every so often, unfortunately, looking more like a dodgy conga dance than any masterpiece!

Another part of our charade was the process of twenty-one people in charge of their own laundry. Allocated laundry days sounded fine in practice but would frequently descend into chaos as people would abandon their washing. Some would be left wet in the machines whilst other items would be half heartedly and ineffectively pegged to the lines, with some owners seeming to abandon any responsibility. Other residents, however, took pride in their belongings and their organisation which would be regularly disrupted by the less thoughtful, who would not think twice at scooping up an armful of clean warm linen from the walk in drying room if it looked vaguely like theirs, much to the utter heartache of Geraldine. So frequently she would lose her freshly washed bedding. She would openly and loudly lose her temper, crying at the top of her voice "Who's got my pigging sheets?" She would be annoyed to the point of distraction and would absolutely insist that each resident, one by one, accompany her to their bedrooms where she would rifle through their drawers and cupboards, look under beds and generally tear the room apart in search of her beloved sheets. It had to be said that almost always they were neatly packed away in the kitchen linen cupboard! Other residents were so tolerating that they would oblige in letting Geraldine search their rooms! Occasionally, she would gain a new necklace or something, whilst on her rounds stating in a broad Lancashire accent "Ain't that necklace loovaly, can I 'av it?" This ultimately meant she forgot about the sacred sheets for a minute or two, not for long however.

Despite the constant attention from staff, management, students and residents the linen cupboard defeated all efforts of achieving any semblance of order!

Throughout the workings of the Mill a balance needed to be struck between the freedom of choice and the imposing of order. It was difficult at times to find an appropriate compromise for some people who would be stuck in their ways. For many reasons people would hoard, collect and find security in their belongings usually because of severe deprivation in earlier life. A sympathetic approach was needed. Mr. T could be seen as one of our challenges. He had an extreme habit of 'collecting' bottles of tomato sauce, vinegar, squash etc. that he bought from the local shop at any opportunity, and when we say an extreme habit, we're talking stacks and stacks of these items barely fitting into his bedroom at times! Helen, being a bit of a softie at times, would buy the ketchup etc. from Mr. T and manage to persuade him to halve his loot, usually paying double the price that they were worth, and put them into the pantry for the house to use (bear in mind Mr. T had had them so long that they were often out of date). Helen would then get told off by Maureen as Terry would use his 'deal money' to buy more ketchup from the shop, hence the problem starting from scratch again.

Thursday

There was a time when Thursday meant tea dancing lessons. A man and his wife would come and teach all those interested how to move on a dance floor! Residents involved could learn to cha cha or foxtrot. Around the same time as the lessons a couple living at the Mill were getting married and the lucky dancers decided to 'train' hard and perform a dance at the reception in front of many guests, and so the tutors began coming on a Thursday night just to train for the reception at which a wedding march would be demonstrated. This caused a lot of excitement among the tea dance bunch. There were just two problems. One older lady would become very 'put out' if she could not dance with the male tutor. Of course he couldn't always dance with her because she had to show moves with his wife and dance partner. This occasionally left this lady huffing and puffing in a corner somewhere. The other trouble was that Mr. T liked to sit in the conservatory where the practice took place and so he would walk through the line of dancers constantly disrupting the class by shouting things like 'gis a fight' or 'Tommy, Ronnie, blue train, with ten bottles of ginger beer on top of his head' or other 'Mr. T phrases'. Such eccentricity was not unusual at the Mill and so long as individuals respected each other, little heed was paid.

Events and activities would vary from week to week, but you could always guarantee that something would happen every single day. There were so many daily dramas and escapades to deal with that they became the norm and few acts or events were surprising! In fact most things in the end were absolutely hilarious!

Humour was the vital key at the mill. Disastrous incidents and bizarre goings on usually ended in laughter and smiles by all and it was that that made the Mill work so well and its uniqueness and style were admired by so many.

There were quite a few pets at the mill over the years, including a beautiful cat called Bailey. He was loved and adored and cared for excellently by Edna. Unfortunately Bailey was hit by a car and died. Edna was understandably devastated.

Because we were such a close knit community sad events would affect everybody on some level. One resident decided kindly that a proper funeral should take place for Bailey – so he kitted himself out in his old choir boy outfit, brought down his electric keyboard and set himself up in the garden, and so the funeral began. He spoke the words of a true vicar, thanked God for Bailey's life with all attendees looking to the floor and feeling sad. Edna at this point was covering her face, trying not to burst into fits of giggles as, very seriously, our locum was giving a funeral fit for royalty. At the end of the service he turned on his keyboard and, slightly out of tune, began playing 'The Old Rugged Cross' which in turn the mourners sang with gusto. By this point Edna and most of the staff and residents were finding themselves with intense belly ache as they tried so desperately not to laugh. Our locum was so intense in his role as a vicar that you could almost imagine him healing the sick with the power of his keyboard! (As you can see, no situation passed without ceremony!).

Friday

Friday equalled pay day. This was a really good thing, but also a disruptive thing. Money was handed out after breakfast. Some residents would wait for the first bus into town to get their essentials, hunt around charity shops or have a quick coffee with a friend. After many discussions at house meetings and staff meetings a drinking ban on Mill premises was imposed. Rules were always reluctantly established as our overall belief system was that people should be given freedom of choice, and although we couldn't prevent people drinking alcohol outside the Mill the disruption it caused made intervention necessary. Almost weekly the ever sweet Maisie would ask someone to help pack her room up, ready for a move. "Dave thinks it's time I had a change" she would comment. "Yes," he said, "Maisie, why don't you move to Sheringham (or Downham or Holt)? You can have a little dog, you know". Of course Dave would have no recollection of these conversations, simply because they didn't take place. Even so, someone was always convinced by her and occasionally would help pack her room (and then unpack it!) The residents and staff at the Mill soon caught on, but this didn't include the unsuspecting new residents, guests, or new staff!

Medication is made up in daily pots by the staff, and depending on the individual is given out weekly, daily or sessionally. Maisie would again insist that Dave had had a word with her about her medication, insisting that Dave said she didn't have to take "that muck". She would insist that he told her "Maisie, you didn't have to take it before you came here and so you don't have to take it now. You don't need it". All new members of staff would be informed that, yes, Maisie did need to take her medication, and no, Dave hasn't told her not to take it. So inevitably Maisie would be given her medication which she would then secretly chuck out of her bedroom window into the car park. Well at least until a member of staff found a great pile of red, oblong tablets just below the window of her freshly packed room!

Drinking was soon replaced by Bingo, so many residents enjoyed winning knick-knacks and the kitchen had an air of silence throughout the game as the numbers were called out. It was taken very seriously, and to be honest would be played until everybody had won a prize. This provided happiness and peace to all those playing and all those working!

Saturday

On a Saturday staff would usually clean the cups from the night before – the dreaded cups that nobody ever washed before going to bed, and usually there would be a sink full waiting!

There was no set time for residents to get up at the weekend, but I usually went off to Swaffham market and took whoever wanted to join me. A jumble sale in the assembly rooms was always our first port of call. A cup of tea and a cake made by the WI was eagerly had by all. In fact Mr T and Andrew would be on their third cup waiting for the rest of us to finish our bargain hunt. We loved it. Most of our residents had very little money and this was a great place to stock up on things for the wardrobe. We collected bits and bobs for others in the house who couldn't scrape themselves out of bed. Peter was one of my favourite people to go on a rummage with. He would go to the auction on the square and come back with some real bargains. We drove Dave mad. "Oh no, what crap have you bought now" he would say. Once Peter purchased a bike. He tied it to the minibus roof rack only for it to come crashing to the floor as we squeezed under the height restricted bar in the car park we were leaving! Gwen was our staff driver then, and she was less than impressed! Peter and I have had gates, chairs, pots, furnishings etc. from our bargain hunts. On one trip from Fakenham everyone had a pot on their laps all the way home. It was the only way we could get them in. We would all be laughing, usually at Dave's expense, as we carted yet more junk home. My trips usually entailed a bit of action. We would have a bag of chips in the bus to eat on the way home. Although my income allowed me to purchase more expensive items I would never create a 'them and us' feeling and was more than delighted to come home with a bargain. I so enjoyed our trips out, and there was even a sing-song on the way home most times!

Sunday

A car boot sale, a trip to our beach hut, or a slob in front of a film on TV were typical activities for a Sunday. I would always take willing participants for a walk – I was incapable of staying indoors all day, whatever the weather. In fact I would love nothing more than a beachcomb or bracing the wind and rain and getting home and sitting in front of the wood burner. I think it helped us all feel alive.

The Sunday roast was always a favourite. Some of the younger residents who enjoyed being left in their beds would be given a call when the Yorkshire puddings went in the oven and usually managed to arrive for 'dish up'. The summer months would often incorporate a BBQ instead.

We always felt that routines were important to living. The challenge for us at the Mill was to create a structure where people felt safe, but not to create institutionalisation. To wake up in the morning and not have a purpose to every day can be soul destroying. We all need a reason to 'be', in order to motivate ourselves and have a sense of direction in life. Obviously this is pertinent to the individual; some people need to fill every minute whilst for others a looser schedule is sufficient for their well being.

Here is a young woman's story in her own words who took her routines to extremes and for whom structure became a destructive obsession. In this as in other similar cases we would work hard to create a feeling of safety and belonging which provided a framework for healthier living.

Living with an eating disorder – a young resident reflects:

4.30 am. I'm up and ready for work which starts at 7am. I am walking there this morning as I do each day, come rain or shine. It used to take me 2.5 hours to walk there, now it takes just 1.5 hours.

Now I must think, I have two rules these days which I mustn't forget – the first rule being not sitting down until 8pm each evening (unless on the exercise bike) and two, eat just one slim-a-soup today. It shouldn't be hard. I've done it for months now, walking at least 10 miles a day.

I weigh five stone eight pounds but I'm still not happy. Another half stone should do it, I will stop then. I am in total control of my life, made increasingly better with each pound I lose. I do two aerobics videos a day (at home) and have six cleaning jobs. I have given up one of my two college courses because I have to sit down for at least two hours at a time. I simply cannot ruin my plans and disobey the rules I have set for myself.

This is my mission in life. I do not need anybody else. It doesn't matter that I have no friends; they would only ruin my routine anyway.

Something is changing today. I wake up hungry, with a hunger so bad that I can't resist. I binge – gorging on all the foods I have been denying myself for months. I can't get enough. I feel possessed, uncontrollably eating anything I can get my hands on; frozen food, out of date food – it doesn't matter.

Now I feel sick, the sickest I have ever felt. I do not feel in control any more. Now I can see myself as I really am – a failure. I try to make myself sick. It doesn't work. This is it. My life is over; I would rather die than be fat. I take an overdose, something I've never really thought about before – why should I? I have been in complete control for months.

The best thing has just happened; I have just had my stomach pumped. The doctors didn't believe I had eaten anything. Just look at their faces now – 5 bucketfuls of vomit later.

I didn't expect this, but then I didn't expect to binge. My rules have now changed. On the days that I binge, I take an overdose, and get my stomach pumped.

My life is a mess. I have limited control and my weight is going up.   Maybe I do need friends after all.

Within myself my fears confined
My own heart set against my own mind
No amount of help can change my ways
No amount of love can heal my days
A lost soul drifting further away
A wasted life never to see brighter days
What went wrong? Who can tell?
The end result: an empty shell
No feelings of love, security and hope
Just feelings of tiredness, helplessness, can't cope
No future to be found, it's just too late
Happiness is not to be, just isn't my fate
An evil life matching an evil person
Impossible to help. Just leave to worsen

CHAPTER ELEVEN

Introduction to Personal Stories

I wanted to include residents' own stories in this book because I feel this reflects how things used to be. I have used a tape recorder and have taken notes. I have kept the words as near as I can to their own words and expressions. All of the residents are aware that I intend to have this book published and will include what they are willing for any member of the public to read. Some residents have kept their own names and identities and some have chosen names for themselves. The stories, to my knowledge, are true. I read them myself and cruised through them as if they were fiction. However, the astonishing lives that some of these lovely folk have had are not fiction and are therefore hard to digest. The next few chapters will give readers an opportunity to read the stories of some of the residents who have passed through the Mill on their journey to recovery.

My name is Roo but that doesn't really tell you who I am. In order to know me you need to know my story.
At six weeks old I was taken into care, along with my sister. We stayed with many foster families but in the end we were sadly split up; my sister went to Norwich and I went to live in Dersingham with my new family who said they had picked me because they wanted me but time would tell that nothing could have been further from the truth. I remember the journey from Norwich. I was travel sick all down my favourite coat and they wouldn't even try and get it clean. I loved that coat, it was black with gold toggles and it was like a comfort blanket to me. They just threw it in the rubbish bin. My foster parents said that Debbie my sister could visit once a fortnight because we didn't want to be separated but Debbie kept running away from her foster home to be with me and we kept phoning each other. Eventually her foster parents put her in a private school and we were banned from phoning each other, so we lost contact. All we

had wanted was to be together but the 'powers that be' said "no". When we were finally parted we screamed and they had to drag us apart. They locked me in the house and forced Debbie into the car. After she had gone there was no comfort given, I was just expected to get on with it.

I had a Social Worker who used to bring me sweets and visit me at school about once a month. I used to tell him I didn't feel wanted, that I didn't fit in. I felt different and upset because the people I was living with didn't want me; they already had three girls of their own. I kept telling him I was unhappy, but all he said was to give it time, that things would settle down. But they didn't. Then he left.

My foster parents treated me totally differently to their own kids. They took their own kids to America and places like that, but even though they went for a month they just left me with neighbours. I was nine when they went to America. They did let me come to Wales with them but I was travel sick on the way and I got the hiding of my life for that. During that holiday whenever they went out they would leave me in the tent. From the age of seven I was abused physically and sexually. I felt I had no-one to turn to. Every night I was the first to have to go up to bed. I was regularly raped. My foster mother knew what was going on; the whole family knew but they did nothing. As a result of what happened my bladder and bowels are permanently damaged and I have been left incontinent. That family told me that because I was a foster child they could do to me what they liked when they liked and they did. I asked for a female Social Worker but they sent a man. I did try to tell him what was going on but whenever he came they would act like the ideal family and pretend that I was the best and most wanted child that ever existed for them.
I lived in terror and began to inflict harm on myself; I cut and burnt myself. I so wanted to die. The school called the NSPCC once but nothing was done about it.

I would bunk off school and I had very few friends. I felt so different, so alone, like I had this terrible sickness that I couldn't tell anyone about. I think if I had told anyone he would have

*killed me. My foster mum's brother and father were abusing me
as well. She would go out shopping and they would come round
and they'd take it in turns to have sex with me. I couldn't bear it.
I'd shut my eyes and pretend I was on this island on my own
because that was the only way I could get through it. They were
all in it together. They would say I was getting what I deserved,
that I encouraged it and that it was my fault. They came to the
house quite frequently, or she would send me to her father's
house and he would do it there. He would say to me "If I buy you
a nice big present what would you do for me?" I knew what he
meant. It was a case of what he would do to me if I didn't have
sex with him. There was never a choice; I just did what I had to
do to survive.*

*Once I told my foster dad that I was going to the social workers
to beg them to come and get me and take me out of this house.
He killed my pet rabbit and said that this was what would
happen to me if I told anyone. Everyone in the neighbourhood
thought they were a marvellous family but behind doors it was a
different matter.*

*On my eighteenth birthday I was moved into a half way house
and gained employment as a cleaner in the Golden Lion Hotel. I
was soon to appear in court and was put on probation for
stealing because I wasn't able to 'make ends meet'. I overdosed
because I couldn't bear people knowing what I'd done. I was
rushed to hospital and put in intensive care. When I came to my
Social Worker was there. Years later I had a meeting with him
and he couldn't understand why I was so angry with Social
Services. When I told him my story he said that he had thought
there was something wrong but that he couldn't put his finger on
it. He said he was sorry. Social Services offered me £250 to
have six therapy sessions as if that would sort me out, but I knew
the damage was done and I couldn't have trusted anyone. I
thought my life was worth more than £250 so I told them to stick
it.*

*I have been given a diagnosis by a psychiatrist; they say I am a
Hebephrenic Schizophrenic. They took me to a specialist unit in*

Birmingham and told me I was just going to look around, but when I got there I had to do a three hour test with no fag breaks or anything. Then they said I shouldn't be allowed near knives and that normally they would look for a long term placement for me at the unit. I refused and stayed at The Mill and went to college to study cooking; they said I was hard working, responsible, very sociable and polite. I qualified while I was at the Mill. I used to study English in the evenings. That shows everyone who said I'd never do anything and who had written me off. I do take medication – it helps keep me stable and allows me to have a quality of life.

I moved on from The Mill and for three years I worked with people who had learning disabilities. I enjoyed using my new found cooking skills and felt valued.

I left work when I became pregnant with my daughter. The father used to beat me up and when she was born he threatened to kill me, so me and my baby went back and stayed at The Mill. I had rung Dave up in tears, desperate to get out of Lynn because I was frightened for my and my daughter's safety. I didn't want him to hurt her. I took him to court and I got custody of my baby. He went off with a fifteen year old and has nothing more to do with us.

My daughter had her own problems. Unfortunately she had serious feeding problems and spent a year and a half in and out of hospital. She couldn't tolerate dairy products and had to be fed through a tube. We had to hold her down and she would scream and scream but we had to do it to keep her alive. She would wet the bed as well. Wet bed, wet clothes, wet everything. Half the time I wasn't getting any sleep. I didn't know what to do; I tried, I really tried, but I just couldn't cope and I went to the nurse and asked for help. They put my child in foster care and I went into the Fermoy Unit for six weeks. Everything soon went pear shaped. I just wanted to rest. A three year battle commenced and Tamara was adopted. I didn't want this to happen. I felt bad. I had hit her round the head.

In Roo's case her life as a child had been stolen. However much the Mill and others put into her as an adult there was so much damage done to her that there would always be a void that could not be filled. I missed her when she left. She was a great cook, she could always make us laugh. Remarkably she managed a good relationship with Dave and they would spend many hours together 'chewing the cud'. She was also my evening partner at Scrabble and we had very competitive games. Roo still has a smile on her face and I am delighted that she is married to a very kind chap. She still has contact with her daughter and we keep in touch occasionally.

Unfortunately it could be very difficult, at times, to work with people who have had such a difficult background. Trust, as you can imagine, was an issue and we as a staff team would have to work hard to gain a trusting and workable relationship to meet the needs of the resident. It took time but the outcomes would be more positive.

We found some residents who had been abused or mistreated in any way often blamed themselves and believed they were the cause of abuse. This could then mean that some would become self destructive and display self harming behaviours and ideas.

Everybody came with a past. We saw a lot of young people pass through our doors, some with past drug problems, others on self destruct. It wasn't just the young, however, that we catered for. Some of our residents had been married, had children, and held down demanding jobs. As I will always say, mental health does not discriminate. Next is Lenny's story. He is a kind, older gentleman who we had the pleasure to work with.

Lenny has a son who suffers with schizophrenia and he also suffers with the condition himself. Lenny's wife died when Andrew was in his late twenties. From then on life became chaotic and out of control. Andrew believed himself to be a talented actor and musician and insisted that Lenny drive him around the country to get work. If Lenny refused Andrew would become violent. He smashed everything up in his home, including light fittings and a television. Lenny lived in terror until one day he collapsed. He was admitted into hospital with delusions and was emaciated due to having no memory to feed himself. Andrew refused any mental health treatment but was sometimes sectioned under the Mental Health Act. Police would at times be called to their house to help with Andrew as he was out of control. His deluded ideas would lead him to believe there were people outside the house waiting to break in and attack him.

Lenny was moved to the Mill by Maggie Devine, a social worker who he will never forget for her concern and kindness. Andrew's life continued to be out of control; he was evicted from their house and became a nomad. He sees himself as a 'street entertainer' and his delusions no longer allow him to acknowledge Lenny as his father. This has been very hard for Lenny to accept although he realized that Andrew is an untreated schizophrenic who has no sense of what reality is and is led by his deluded thought patterns.

At times Lenny's own voices frighten and disturb him. His illness has led him to believe that various people have come into his room. Once a group of Russians came in, on another occasion people came to taunt him. He described wanting to get a gun and shoot them. Lenny tells how one night a policeman turned up and started pulling on him; "It woke me up" he said. "My mother's voice has visited me amongst other nice voices, I like listening to them". Lenny has a slow release depot injection that helps keep his unwanted voices out of his head. Whilst at the Mill he decided to stop having the injection but sadly frightening voices soon returned and the medication had to be resumed. He brought his dog Lucky to live with him at the Mill. Lucky was eighteen years old, blind, nearly bald and incontinent. They loved each other until the day Lucky died. Lenny now has a new dog called Sam.

Lenny had permission to drive the company's car which he loved as he said it gave him freedom and space. He was often seen taking my sons, Shane and Lee, into town with him.

He is a true gentleman and I feel so pleased that this lovely man shared so many good experiences with us and his life was enriched by us giving him a place to live where he felt safe and cared for.

Next is an account of how one resident lived with the effects of bi-polar disorder, an illness which can be so difficult to live with.

I am flying high, soaring above the eagles. I have been up since 4am and have been spinning like a top. Floors have been mopped, dishes done and now I await you eagerly to announce that I have BAKED YOU A PIE! I have never been so happy in all my life, so full of joyous ecstasy. I want to shop and buy beautiful presents for all the poor people and everyone. I want to talk and talk until no words are left. I will talk with God for I am high and lifted. If I seek him and fast for forty days and nights then he will gather me up and angels will talk to me. I will know mysteries because I am a prophetess and God has given me a message for this nation. Woe to those who will not listen or pour scorn on me. They plot against me, seeking to silence a servant of God.

Oh God, let my life on earth end. I am a useless sinner, a failure, a Pharisee. I don't want my life, take me to you, intervene merciful Father and let me come into your kingdom. You will judge me and beat me so surely I should long for old age but I don't. I mean nothing; my life is meaningless and futile. Why can't I work and have a mortgage? I know I am not fit to have a family. My brothers and sister don't let me change their children's nappies. They must think I am a paedophile. Maybe they are right, maybe they sense something I don't. I am the worst kind of scum, I hate myself, I should be punished. I know I am capable of terrible things - of murder. Sleep - I must sleep, I need sleep. I will take my tablets and try to sleep, make it all go away.

I will see someone today. I will feel better today - don't go up town or read, keep it nice and quiet. You'll be okay. Pray for peace, ask for mercy and be thankful. You have survived, you

*would have regretted death by your own hand. It will be okay
again.*

We had so many wonderful characters at the Mill. Over time
people came and went. I must say how brave I found new
residents. To come (usually from a hospital setting) and find
their niche within our community, could, I imagine be very
difficult. Some would find the transition period very difficult
and equally some would feel at home straight away. Fez
describes how she felt at the prospect at living at the Mill and the
reality of it.

*I had been in the mental health care system for one year and I
was supposed to be ready for independent living, but had found
myself back in hospital. My social worker Joy came to visit me,
she was very animated, saying "we have found somewhere suited
to you, the best place!" She continued, so very excited, saying
that there was an alternative place in North Norfolk, like a
commune, full of amazing people. Everybody had really good
outlooks, she said, and everyone mucks in and it sounds fun. It
sounded too good to be true so I enthusiastically agreed to visit,
full of hope and feeling lucky; (a) I had such a good social
worker who cared about finding somewhere to suit my
personality and (b) this place actually existed here in Norfolk. I
had been used to a home (residential), warm and comfortable
with good support. I couldn't really fault it but it lacked
something that I was later to find in the Mill in Gayton.*

*When I arrived there I was chuffed. It was such a nice old
building. I immediately felt like I was in an actual mini
community under <u>one</u> roof. There were seventeen residents in a
brightly coloured maze of a house with animals (which I later
cared for and loved). It was so homely, the people seemed to all
respect where they were (with good vibes) and looked like they
were holding onto a secret, which I was later to discover to be
the Millers' philosophy; the common bond between us and of
being valued by each other, the workers and especially the
owners. The owners' infectious humour and outlook was to be so
contagious. It was like we were all being in on one big joke and*

getting it, and that being at the start of recovery, the feeling of somewhere not taking mental health issues seriously with all the doom and gloom that comes with it was somewhere to start.

Later I'd find myself singing songs I'd learnt whilst washing up, expressing myself through clothes people gave me which I loved (from workers and other residents), eating good wholesome food which we cooked and shared, going camping, horse riding, meeting really cool people, making friends, going on brilliant holidays, laughing lots, gardening, meetings, Christmas never to forget, voluntary work and so much more. All of these would be routes to happiness, all kinds were catered for and so everyone was bound to find something for themselves and of course I found several of my own.

The owners, Helen and Dave, were always completely consistent and utterly reliable, something which to me seemed almost superhuman. I feel even today I value that attitude and try to copy it. In the turmoil of mental illness that can be invaluable. The illness was just something that happened whilst living the Millers life and it was encouraged to take a back seat; lucky for me, as if I had been anywhere else the illness would have consumed me. I know this because I left the Mill after seven years to attempt independent living. Living in a flat close to my parents, it did consume me for a while. I tried living with two other people, thinking maybe that it was living alone that caused this, but things didn't improve, so I returned to the Mill and gradually my illness took a back seat again.

Funny stories from Fez:

All of us were down in the dumps sometimes. So Helen suggested we all take the dogs down to Bawsey, a nearby beauty spot with lakes and woods and sand dunes. We wandered around aimlessly until we came to a hill. Helen shouted "Go on then! Run! Run down!". We all careered down the sandy slope and were soon laughing and exhilarated, our woes forgotten. The best therapy ever!

A group of us once went to the Costa Brava in Spain. Dave and Netty, Karen, Ray, Frances, Dulcie, Serena, Johnny and me were sitting on the porch one evening having a tipple of the extremely cheap booze, chilling out. A few annoying ants (which were everywhere) marched by. Dave said "I didn't anticipate that", then as a few more marched by Netty said "How anti social" then the "antagonising truth". This ant joke lasted the whole holiday, as long as the garlic mayonnaise stuff in a jar, called 'Aioli', which we had on everything. Tee hee.

On the same holiday a lovely elderly lady called Dulcie was paddling in the sea and a larger than anticipated wave broke and she slipped and fell. A group of people came to her rescue and called out to Dave "Your mother has fallen in the sea!" We laughed and Dave looked a little perplexed. We joked about it for the rest of the holiday!

One day we went on a day trip to Blakeney Point, a popular tourist place where you can see basking seals. We all got in an open wooden boat and motored out to the Point. On the way we saw a tree growing out of the sea; it was so surreal and bizarre that my close friend Sarah and I were in stitches. Like a Monty Python sketch, this set the tone for our trip. We approached the basking seals and were still laughing when Sarah said "Imagine if we were all at the Mill doing our stuff and all those seals went on a trip to look at us!" She had a point and we giggled and watched the seals, quite bemused.

On one of our many holidays to Derbyshire where we were known to walk miles (all the exercise did wonders for our mental state). We went to these caves which had boats underground from which you could view them. We all put on our helmets and Dave sang "Hi ho, hi ho, it's off to work we go!" There were a hundred steps to go down in a kind of tunnel. I went down ten and started to panic, I was sort of claustrophobic, and ran back up followed by my friend, Sarah, as I had spooked her. We bottled out but the others really enjoyed it.

The Mill was always the place for song; often we sang and it was the done thing to join in. Lots of us were members of a choir or had enjoyed visits by the choir on an afternoon. Singing made light of big washing and drying up for seventeen people. Of an evening, Sarah and I would sit at the table and sing a universal song as we both enjoyed travelling people in our lives. We really loved how we felt after this song; it truly lifted our spirits.

When I arrived at the Mill I couldn't believe I was permitted to keep my cat and was put in a room with a cat flap. Animals are so healing. The Mill also had dogs which we loved and cared for. We saw animals come and go; my cat got run over. Everyone was so kind and we even had a proper little burial with a prayer from my friend, Karen. This was so important to me, and these sort of important events were always happening for people which is how it should be.

I used to be a staff nurse and I am now a volunteer at the local hospital. I really enjoy my role and I believe I have a much greater understanding having been unwell and vulnerable myself.

Now I'm living very happily in an outreach house; being valued and encouraged is the magic here. I have through the years made many friends and friends of friends and friends of friends of friends, due to community spirit, and this has made me feel at home and accepted. I never imagined this when I first went to hospital and was diagnosed because of the stigma around mental illness.

Sadie, happily married with three children, gives a reflection of her time at the Mill:

The Mill kitchen was always the centre of daily activity. Socially, food was extremely important to everyone. On my first day I was left on my own to make tea for fourteen. Initially daunted, it didn't take long to fathom that you couldn't go wrong with Shepherd's Pie.

Helen would feed people with just about everything going. She was a master at shopping for her extended family and we all learnt to hone in on yellow labels, because yellow meant cheap and we liked cheap. She was also good at not wasting anything. Sunday you would see the Sunday roast, Monday the leftovers would be covered in cheese sauce and presented as a vegetable bake. In fact people will eat just about anything if you cover it in a sauce, and this was the case when Helen made Game Pie. Some of us who had the nod stayed well clear. It could have been road kill for all we knew...no one complained though and thought the 'chicken' pie tasted good.

If curry or chilli had been on the menu one evening the chances were someone, normally accompanied by Helen, would be eating it for breakfast the following day.

The larder cupboard grew over the years as more people joined the throng. As I said previously, yellow labels were always rife and half the tins would be out of date, but hey, no one died; besides, most of them had tried to kill themselves already!

Horse riding

Helen loved to ride and she was good, and so as one of our recreational activities we would go riding. The only experience of riding most of us had had was on a merry go round. Horses seem to sense when you know very little. I sat on one and the stable hand said that I should be in the yard. I pointed out that I knew this, but the horse had other ideas as it munched flowers on the roadside. We would walk along the beach, some trotting, others begging the person who was leading them not to let go. The next day we would walk as if still sitting on horseback because our muscles felt that fused.

One of the funniest horse riding jaunts was on a trip to Derbyshire. Donna, our little starlet, said she had ridden before. So as the rain drizzled down she mounted her steed. The trouble was it was an ex race horse who had a fear of water. The horse decided to gallop off half way round with Donna's little legs bouncing rapidly at the horse's sides.

Derbyshire

Helen mainly took us on trips, the exception being Derbyshire, which was Dave's baby, being his homeland. He would drive the minibus to probably the most remote cottage in the county. To reach it you had to go down a long track, leaving all signs of civilisation behind. Mod cons were at a minimum, the shower was situated in the shed and if you looked up in the shower you could see daylight or moonlight. The chemical toilet was the job of the men to empty, the females being kitchen based.

CHAPTER TWELVE

Our residents were a mixed bag. At times people would come with very complex needs. People never fit into tidy boxes, therefore a learning disability, physical disability and a mental health problem at times all came together in one person. This would be after the different agencies had finished trying to push the responsibility of the resident onto each other as the responsibility would affect the budget of the organisation deemed to be responsible. The most prominent disability would usually decide what Social Services or NHS camp they ended up in.

JR kindly agreed to enter into a conversation with Helen with a view to it being used as part of this book. This is a painful process for JR, and we are grateful to him for sharing his story and insights for the benefit of others. In JR's own words "I don't like talking about my past, it gives me bad memories". For many people reliving experiences is difficult but can be illuminating for the reader – thank you JR for your courage:

JR's life has been a fight against a string of adversities that began when he was only three when his mother couldn't cope and put him into care. He stayed at the children's home until he was eight and had another unsuccessful spell living with his mother. The placement at home soon broke down and he returned to the children's home where he stayed until the age of sixteen. He was then placed in a flat in his own flat. His day to day life was lived in a muddle dealing with his physical and learning disabilities and mental health problems. He felt abandoned by the professionals and caring systems. Eventually the chaos became too much and he was admitted into the local psychiatric hospital. From there followed many placements in residential care. JR is a man who has strived to pursue his hobbies and interests and he thrives on keeping busy. Many of the residential placements broke down as JR found the environments too sedentary. JR was moved to the Mill for a fresh start, he was given ways to channel his energies into a positive lifestyle. He was coaxed to find alternative outlets for his emotional and mental distress.

It is necessary in telling JR's story to recount a little detail of the physical, emotional and mental hurdles that face him each day. When JR was three he suffered a stroke that affected his left hand, arm and leg. Despite the efforts of a physiotherapy team JR cannot use his left hand and his left arm and leg are shorter than the right. In addition to this one foot is a size 6 and the other a size 9. JR cannot afford to buy two pairs of shoes and doesn't like to waste, so he buys a pair of size 9 and stuffs the toe of one shoe with newspaper to make it fit. To add to this JR has had to contend with a deep burgundy birthmark which is known as a port-wine stain. This covers much of his face, despite skin grafts. JR's eyes, forehead and nose are all affected. He has been the victim of much unkind teasing which used to bother him in his late teens.

JR has learning disabilities and mental health issues, suffering frequently with bouts of depression during which he will tend to self harm. In the past he has taken overdoses, cut himself and poured petrol over himself. With help however JR has learned that even if you feel desperate and down there are other ways out of the situation. Now he knows he has to seek help as soon as he needs it.

JR also has problems controlling his anger, and although he has never been physically violent he realises he can be verbally aggressive. When JR feels down he can find it difficult to even get out of bed, sometimes for days on end. Taking medication can also be difficult during these spells. Swallowing the tablets is an emotional issue as well as a physical one and seems to require energy and will that is missing.

Incorporated in the layout of the Mill is a cottage and at this point in time that is where JR lives. He is now more independent, doing his own menus and shopping, cooking and laundry. There is help from the staff if needed and JR can always ask if he gets stuck. This combination of independence and support gives JR a feeling of self esteem, safety and security.

At the end of the day, however, JR's attitude of self-help has played a significant role in improving his lot in life. He works on an allotment where he can let off steam. He has help and support from staff when cooking and budgeting and he has a motorised bike which allows him freedom of movement. JR's attitude of self help has played a significant role at improving his lot in life. I shall close with a few of JR's own words;
"Coping with depression isn't easy. In my life if I don't keep my mind occupied I get low. If you help yourself, people will help you".
Some valuable words from JR.

There have been some wonderful people pass through our door. I came to be fond of so many and enjoyed working with some great folk! Julian came to us in the early days, and I loved his personality immediately, big, black and beautiful, he was quite simply a star!

Julian came from a warm loving family with one brother. His mum was a very successful woman who worked for local government. Julian had been adopted as a baby and had enjoyed a loving childhood. All went well until his late teens when he started experimenting with drugs and alcohol. It was the beginning of a downhill spiral which he would struggle with for the next few years. Mental health problems kicked in and soon he was admitted into the local psychiatric services. It was to be one of many admissions.

Julian came to live at the Mill House to recover, after living a chaotic lifestyle for the last few years. The locals in the pub loved him and used to call him Tyson. He had been diagnosed with paranoid schizophrenia; a label that didn't seem to fit his character. He laughed from his belly upwards into his large round jolly face with twinkling dark brown eyes. This laugh was infectious to all around him, like a laughing policeman you see at the funfair. He was big and cuddly and oozed warmth and kindness. My boys engaged with him immediately and spent many hours playing games with him and laughing. He was like having a breath of fresh air in the house.

However, he did have a few challenging character traits, munching through the fridge at night where nothing was safe! He could easily snack out on a couple of pounds of sausages. His appetite was insatiable.
He wasn't keen on changing his clothes or having a regular scrub up. His sex drive was always at the ready, and he would appropriately 'sniff' out any willing participant. One day I thought I could hear a baby upstairs. As I listened more closely, I could hear a baby, it was making gurgling noises and the sound was coming from the bathroom. I gingerly pushed the door back and there in the bath in a makeshift cosy bed was a beautiful baby. Julian's room was opposite this communal bathroom. There was only one place for the mother to be. I said "Julian, there seems to be a baby in the bath. Do you happen to know where its mother is"? A Julian roar of laughter came from the other side of the bedroom door. I suggested they might like to come and collect the baby as a communal bathroom was perhaps not the best place to leave it, and others in the house may find it disconcerting and confusing, particularly if they wanted to take a bath.

A small gang of us went to Tunisia together on holiday. I shared with a girl who had OCD and it was fascinating watching her make her bed which consisted of two cotton sheets and a throw and two pillows and to place her small collection of toiletries out on her shelf, and remake the bed that was already made and immaculate. It took her forty minutes; the precision of the process was incredible. She was a lovely person, she had achieved a first at University, had a high powered job, was tall slim and very attractive, but was crippled by her mental health problems. They dictated her life and left her unable to feel content with anything she tried to achieve. Watching her operate with me for the week was such an education. I reflected on her bedroom at the mill. Although it was a no go zone for anybody to step beyond the threshold, I would peep in when she came to the door to receive a message and the carpet which once looked dead and flat now stood with a pert green pile. She had obviously spent many hours grooming the dead carpet back to life. The need for order in her life was astonishing. I asked her once if she wanted to come into Norwich with me. She declined because today was not the day to put on a clean sweatshirt, even though she looked immaculate. If it had of been a clean sweatshirt day she could have come with me.

Back to our holiday and Julian. He became loved by everyone. The waiters at every meal took delight in feeding him. The entertainments manager who organised all sorts of family dressing up games and competitions enjoyed him as he was up for everything. Lee my son who was ten at the time couldn't have been away with anybody more entertaining although it did annoy him that Julian would lie in bed too often. He was usually sleeping off his consumption of too much food and drink. The beach security guard seemed to like us, giving us lots of non verbal communication. It could have had something to do with me being nearly six months pregnant and wearing only bikini knickers. Julian would lie next to me on the beach; we must have looked like a couple of beached whales!

One day when we had left the safety of our private beach and taken a stroll into town along a long sandy beach we stopped for a camel ride. (Sorry Dave, I did promise not to ride a camel while pregnant or do anything silly.) The men with the camels were a bit "rough round the edges" to say the least. They took up quite a fascination with me, and clearly thought Julian was my partner. Apparently a pregnant woman was quite desirable and they were negotiating, or trying to talk Julian into giving me away for a camel or two. His belly laughter alerted me to something 'fishy' going on and I suggested we moved on. The rest of the week he threatened me with camel trade if I 'nagged' him.

We enjoyed the amateur dramatic group together in Kings Lynn. Again Julian became the star of the show, not because he took the lead role, but because he was so charismatic. The director and cast loved him. The performance went on for a few days at the Arts Centre, mostly achieving full house audience. We had such fun and quality time together.

Having achieved some drama experience, we decided that Julian would play baby Jesus in the Mill pantomime this particular Christmas. The excitement of the role was all too much, so he went to the local and calmed himself with a few beers. The house was buzzing, cooking and making a feast for the evening. The crowd was normally over a hundred. Annette, who was a great cook and had made some delicious looking trays of quiche to be cut into squares for the party feast that evening, had them cooling on the kitchen side when Julian arrived back from his light refreshments from the pub. He had yet again over indulged himself and as he tripped up the kitchen step he projectile vomited across the top of the quiche. All of our faces must have looked a picture. Annette said loudly 'Julian'. His response was a smile and he said "It's all right Netty, you can just wash the top off, no harm done"! The quiche was binned with disgust.

There was a serious side to Julian and to this day I can feel the intense sensitivity of feeling when he would talk to me about the energy it took for him to re-establish himself after a breakdown. Twice he had got himself a flat, girlfriend and a feeling of safety and comfort when the 'slippery slope' of deteriorating mental health would start to creep upon him. His thoughts would become bizarre, he would lose his reality of the world. He told me he once dressed up as a jester with a woman's dress on, Airware boots, and jester's hat and went into a building society and said 'It's a hold up – give me all your money'. The girl at the desk, not taking him seriously, said 'Do you want the cheques?' He replied 'Yes, make them out to Julian Rostrum". Needless to say he was arrested and put into hospital.

He said "I haven't got the energy to keep rebuilding my life", after an episode of frightening, bizarre and wearing illness. On one occasion we worked hard at avoiding a hospital admission. His behaviour was chaotic; he lit candles up each stair of our house to stop us being harmed. He covered the floor with newspapers. He wanted to take my boys away to give them new musical experiences. He was very high maintenance and eventually, and very sadly, he was admitted under Section 3 of the Mental Health Act. We eventually called in services after we found a tie hanging in the tree in the garden. Fortunately the branch had broken and Julian was still alive. His safety was clearly at risk, therefore we had no choice. On this occasion life became more and more disturbing, the local psychiatric ward were intimidated by him and found his behaviour too much to handle. Eventually he was placed in a secure hospital in Norwich. His determination to end his life was achieved by hanging himself in the summer house in the grounds.

The sadness was immense for so many. However, having had the true Julian talk to me I could understand his reason. He had lost his energy to fight for survival. My only consolation was the feeling of peace for him.

Having been such a fun loving colourful character, the funeral was upbeat. We took the mini bus full of staff and residents. Chris, who found it difficult to go anywhere without a pack up and flask of coffee, started munching and had poured himself a cup of coffee before we had even got outside the Mill gateway. It made me smile; Julian would have loved it and most certainly joined in with a sandwich. The congregation were every shape and size, middle class, working class, unemployed, hippies, the majority looking as if they were off to a festival, an appropriate crowd to say goodbye to a glorious character.

It was great to see residents on their journey to recovery. I would watch with admiration and pride as people grew into being self sufficient, and independent. It was a good feeling to see residents move on from the Mill. But it was distressing to find that, because of limited resources in the 'system' those 'going it alone' found it so, so difficult and sometimes impossible. Residents would be living with us in our little community, surrounded by people day in and day out. It was great that some wanted to gain independence and we embraced this wholeheartedly. But there was no Most residents moved straight from the Mill and into a flat of their own and it would become too much too soon. We saw this happen so much that we decided to open semi-independent houses whereby staff would spend time each day with the occupants to continue support with the aim of encouraging further independence.

Below is a story of a lady's journey after leaving Mill House;

"When I first arrived at the Mill and during those first heady months I thought that I would live there forever. However even the most idyllic settings can wear thin with time and familiarity and after about two and a half years I was setting my sights on a move back to independence. The opportunity came up for a two bed roomed housing association flat.

I handed in the necessary months notice and started filling in forms and speaking to social workers and Julian Housing support workers. I would see someone for half an hour once a week. This was a big drop from the twenty four hour support. As my leaving date approached I began to realise that I had considered everything but my mental health. Panic set in and I closed down. I would sit in my pyjamas all day not talking, not eating. I had passed the point of no return and suddenly I felt that the loss of the Mill was becoming one massive bereavement.

And so it was with massive misgivings that I moved into that which I had so eagerly sought - a flat of my own. I sat there on my own the day I moved in. My support worker had left, and I was surrounded with boxes and bags but not an ounce of enthusiasm. In the end Helen sent a manic resident down to help me and she cleaned the cupboards, emptied the boxes and made up my bed.

I lived in a state of terror. During the spring and summer months I would sit up all night until dawn broke before snatching a few hours sleep. Before long the situation had deteriorated so that I wouldn't bath or shower, listen to music or watch the television for fear that someone might break in without me hearing. My dosage of sedation was through the roof but such was my fear, however exaggerated it might seem, that the adrenalin just counteracted all medical attempts to help me relax. Desperate and with no escape I made an attempt at killing myself. Although I was very ill, I didn't die and at least the mental health team realised this wasn't a workable situation. I was referred back to the waiting list for the Mill, much to my relief, and moved back in about four months later.

CHAPTER THIRTEEN

Powers tells his story

I'm 31 years old. I was sectioned under the Mental Health Act after spending time in prison where it was deemed I needed hospitalization and was moved to the Norvic Clinic. In all I was locked up for five years. I have never understood why. I'm still under restrictions with the Home Office but I lead a normal life these days.

I feel that as a young man I have become a target for society's fear. I have an interest in martial arts. In my early twenties I spent a lot of time in psychiatric hospitals after living on the streets when my parents moved to Wales. After a fight with a Big Issue seller I was put in seclusion in Hellesdon Hospital. It was very irritating being watched all the time and on one of these occasions I punched a male nurse in the face. I couldn't stand him watching me any longer. I was placed in a semi secure unit which was part of Hellesdon Hospital. That was my first experience of a punitive system. Later I was arrested for carrying a Samurai sword which led to a prison sentence, which I found very hard. I was taking prescribed medication and locked up for twenty two hours a day. I started smoking for something to do and each week I spent my £2.50 allowance on tobacco. I was given medication that made me vomit and interrupted my eating and sleeping patterns. I now take a drug with no side effects. Doctors insist that I take it because they think that there is something wrong with the chemicals in my head. I don't agree with them – I don't think there is anything wrong with me. There are things that are out of control in my life as in anybody's life but I don't think the solution is to give someone drugs. I don't want the doctors; I just want to live my life.

My mother was a teacher and my father worked in management. Between the ages of eighteen and nineteen I travelled around India. I needed to be my own person and escape from my family's altruistic values. On my return my parents called the doctor and said "There're some people here who want to talk to you" and that sort of thing. I was manhandled into an ambulance, and given injections for having my own opinion about things. I was really pissed off with my parents. As it was happening to me it felt as if I was in a Hollywood movie. It was so unreal. I feel let down by my brother. He should have taken my side; I'd say it was a brother's job. My sister I can understand - she wouldn't go against my parents. I don't see any of them now. They had me hospitalised so I go it alone now. There are animals in the Serengeti with better family relationships. I made an artistic decision and changed my name from Adam. I needed to be my own person. I may change my name again in the future.

I feel as if I've been treated like some crazy dude rather than someone who has their own spiritual guidance. My own spirit is essentially what gets me through. I think there is ignorance about the way I live my life. Living at the Mill let me be who I am and as far as I am concerned it was a better 'family' than the one I grew up with. I have no respect for medical opinions although I do have a good doctor now. I waited six months for a bed at the Mill. I visited about fifteen times before I moved in. I loved it. Communal life suited me and I like pulling together. That's why I like the Mill. I screwed up on my last visit and thought that I'd blown my chance. I got pissed, threw up on the pub floor and got the whole house banned.

I enjoy writing and art. For many years I called myself an artist; I went to Art College for two weeks before I was expelled. At the Mill I painted a mural on the kitchen wall. It was a copy of an artist I admire called Norma Matthews. I also did a yellow submarine as I love the Beatles; they were a great band. The pictures were twenty foot long by six foot. Most of the staff and residents liked my work. I also painted pictures for the sitting room walls of horses and cavalry. I copied some of Roddy Mattus's work in the laundry room. I loved going to Homebase. I bought paint that you have mixed for specific colours. I was given my favourite bedroom at the back of the house. It overlooks the beautiful garden and summer house. I spend many *hours in the summer house which I painted in bright primary colours. On sunny days I lay in the hammock. It's a more beautiful and realistic way of spending time than being in a locked ward in a hospital. I go to London on visits. I've been taught Tai Chi by Simon for a whole year up at Helen and Dave's home. It's very demanding and physical. I enjoy making a camp fire and cooking sirloin steak. I set up the Sherlock Holmes Hell Fire Club; those who wanted would go to the quiet room where we would listen to sets of CDs we were given, take notes and discuss what we thought of the stories. Thanks Dave and Helen for giving me a break.*

Devistal:

Despite the colour of my skin, and offending at seventeen, I'm now on the right path!

My name is Devistal. I lived in London with my mum, dad, five brothers and three sisters. There was no family harmony, only arguments and violence.

At the age of seventeen I had been involved in street violence and gang warfare. It was this lifestyle that led me to serve many years behind bars. I had stabbed a person. He had been my friend. I felt let down by him and betrayed. I had felt that he had disrespected me. To this day I am still shocked at what I did. I felt peer pressure from the gang to react at what he had done to me and what I felt was self defence at the time led me to kill my old friend with a stab wound.

Prison was hard. I was 25 years old when I came out. I had gained some good things such as education, activities and music. I had been in a detention centre followed by a stay in Wandsworth, Brixton and Wayland prison. I had to grow up fast.

I went to the Mill to live when I left prison. From the day I arrived it felt like déjà vu. I felt as if I belonged there; I felt respected, valued and safe. I was at last able to live with myself. I look back on the times I was bullied, traumatised and anxious. My family had faded away during my years in prison.

Living at the Mill gave me opportunities I couldn't have hoped for living in West London. I had left the concrete jungle and replaced my environment with green fields and the countryside.

The Mill was a healing place to live. People adapted to the behaviour of others. We had a brilliant time cooking, horse riding and bike riding, and they knew how to throw a good party. They knew how to celebrate each other's birthdays and Christmas. Each and every person was accepted for who they were. We were given opportunities to grow up and discover who we were; the Mill was a special place.

When I left the Mill I lodged in town with a friend of Helen and Dave until I was given a council flat. I got a job with a commercial cleaning company and felt confident with my new independent lifestyle. Sadly my happiness didn't last. My flat was in a deprived area. I took a lot of racial abuse from the local children, but this didn't worry me as I had heard it all before. The neighbour above became my new abuser. He objected to the colour of my skin and made my life a misery with his constant intimidation. He was a well known member of a large family who spent a lot of time on the wrong side of the law. My mental health became fragile; anxiety and depression returned to my life. I felt, before I snapped, that I needed to get out. I moved into a flat in a communal house in a lovely village near the Norfolk Broads.

I often think about the years I lived at the Mill and the memories I will never forget. I shall always be grateful to my probation officer for the support she gave me and for facilitating my move to the Mill. I now help out in my new village, acting as a volunteer. I am thankful for the confidence I have gained because I am in a position to give something back to the community I now live in.

Sometimes reports and information would be given to me referring a resident to our care. Regardless of what the information said (and at times this could be quite scary) I always felt the need to meet the person and do my own thorough investigation, including my own natural instincts before declining to take somebody because of their past history. Presentation of written information, I found, could sometimes cloud the real person.

Duncan:

I truly believe that had I not spent the time I did at Community Support Homes my life would be very different. I regard my decision to become a resident as the most important decisions I have ever made.

My life had been a constant barrage of hospital stays, both physical and psychiatric. As I look back reflectively I can see what a nightmare I was. I lacked the insight into what I was doing and the lifestyle I was creating. I used to fight and go out of my way to destroy myself and make other's lives a misery. I look back on this with shame and embarrassment. I spent my youth thinking life was about me and everyone owed me. How wrong I was.

The wakeup call came when I was shown that respect and humility were the keys to success. I have vivid memories of Helen, Dave and many others telling me many things that I had needed to hear for so long. I learned to stand on my own two feet and behave appropriately around other people. Over the seven years of residency I met some very special people who together with my own endeavours turned my life around and changed the way I think forever. The people I met, both residents and staff, still mean a great deal to me.

In hindsight my days as a resident of CSH were the happiest of my young to middle-aged life. A big part of my contentment of living at the Mill was the relationship I built with a cross collie dog called Modeine. I loved that dog and was devastated when she died of old age. To this day I still have her lead and tennis ball. When I look at these good memories come flooding back.

I put in a lot of hard work with my own self development and was helped by many others for which I shall always be grateful. It has been a long, hard road but it is achievable and if my story gets that message across to one person I shall be pleased.

I left CSH's in October 2007. It has not been plain sailing. To be honest I knew that it wouldn't be. I now live in a pretty bungalow with a big garden in a respectable neighbourhood. I am gently moving forward to part time work and I am getting involved in local events. I can now look in the mirror and be proud of who I am.

I am so proud to say that we had so many success stories. Many of our residents didn't perhaps beat their demons, but learnt to live around them and make a life for themselves where they found fulfilment and realised their potential. For some this meant a return to careers and relationships, others achieved an independent lifestyle in the community. Others still found ways in which they could manage their illnesses to a degree that optimised their quality of life.

Ian has managed just that:

I moved into the Mill after living with my loving parents who could no longer cope with my depression and Asperger's Syndrome. I had many admissions to the local psychiatric unit. My anger at times was out of control and I would often be breaking things. The Mill gave me one to one support and soon I felt less isolated. I moved in on the 13th August 2002 on the same day as Nick and we still remain good friends. My parents looked relaxed and stopped worrying, knowing I was getting the support I needed. There was something at the Mill I had never experienced before and that was team work. The staff were great at their jobs.

We felt like a big family and we had good times and bad. On 2nd October 2002 we went to Legoland in Windsor. I'm a big Lego fan and eventually used Lego characters in my graphic design college course. I lived at the Mill for eight months. I enjoyed all the fun we had; Sarah putting tomato ketchup in the rubber gloves used for washing up (poor Evelyn), our egg fight in the kitchen and me dressing up as a baby. I enjoyed my gay social club and playing football and games at the sports hall with

Helen and Dave on a Monday night.

I moved on to live in Norwich, started a college course and gained a distinction in my BTEC national diploma amongst other qualifications. I have had some amazing jobs in design, TV set design, puppet theatre, a story book for children and a lighting company. As I have got older hitting rock bottom has become less frequent, thank God! Depression can grip you like a disease but my Asperger's has given me the strength to move forward and be creative.

CHAPTER FOURTEEN

We always had lots of people pass through the doors in any given day. Social workers, CPN's, friends and family of residents piled in each day. Karen, an ex resident and good friend speaks of our most frequent visitors; workmen;

The Mill was an old building and at times seemed to be determined to malfunction as much as its inhabitants. This led to a constant stream of tradesmen pitting their wits against various antiquated systems.

As with everything else to do with the Mill, the collection of workmen employed to keep the building in working order were certainly colourful.

The most popular visitors were the builders, Wilm and Mitch, two brothers who fitted in well and seemed oblivious to whatever chaos was going on around them. Wilm was married to Maggie Devine, a social worker who favoured an Indian style of dress and exotic jewellery.

When not working, Wilm would also adopt Indian dress. He is tall with long hair and a long beard. The effect I can assure you is quite striking.

Mitch is friendly and fitted in well at the Mill, seeming to enjoy the atmosphere. The two brothers were versatile and industrious, not qualities you could use to describe all the workmen that visited us. One particular character, George, arrived to check the fire safety carrying his guitar. Maureen was impressed with his willingness to engage with the residents and entertain them with his musical arrangements. Several hours later Maureen was less impressed and the residents had beaten a hasty retreat.

Maureen was often a focus for various love sick or lusty workmen who were far more intent on doing some clumsy (and fruitless), flirting rather than fixing the plumbing or wiring in yet another extractor fan.

Mick the electrician worked at the Mill and sister houses for ten years. Here's what he thought of us;

"I loved working at Community Support Homes. There was always a sense of fun around the place and it was never dull. On one occasion I was having a cuppa in the kitchen when one of the lads kept shouting "There goes another one". I asked what he meant and he said "Porsches and Ferraris are going by the window". I went across to look as a Ford Fiesta was passing. "There goes another one". He seemed happy enough, so a bit confused I went back to my cup of tea.
One morning I arrived at the Mill to find a bike on top of the roof. A few minutes later a resident came out and asked if anyone had seen his bike. I said "As it happens I have seen a bike on the roof". He looked up unfazed and said "Yes, that's my bike" like it was normal!
Another time one of the chaps threw a microwave out onto the patio. The staff and residents were unfazed. Apparently the man who was coming to fix it was late, and this chap had a rigid thinking problem.
I also soon learnt not to have my van washed by an eager resident. The first time I paid £1 for a wash. When I returned to my van later I found it covered in mud. I couldn't see out of the window and had to drive to the nearest car wash!
It was a great place to work!

Let's move from maintenance to music. Karen has her say;

I suppose that with Dave and Helen both being of a musical inclination ("It's good for the soul, darling") it was pretty inevitable that music would feature in the life of the Mill.
In actual fact Dave had a band called 'Close Call' which had come into being as a result of a jamming session between a student called John Heley, a resident by the name of Peter, and Dave. With the addition of Graham Hull on guitar and John Paige on drums the outfit was complete. The Millers were loyal fans and Ady had special status as the band's roadie. The band had regular gigs and these would be attended by enthusiastic Millers who would always be keen to strut their stuff on the dance floor. Some of the venues were not the most up market places, and the Queen's Arms definitely comes into this category. On one occasion Dave was singing the opening words to 'Broken

Glass' as a chair came crashing through a glass window, thrown by a disgruntled customer who had been evicted earlier in the evening.

The females of the Mill were not to be out done however. With Helen taking the lead gradually more and more of the female residents joined the Castleacre-based Big Heart and Soul Choir. The choir was itself suitably unconventional and was therefore able to absorb our colourful characters without the blink of an eye. Some choir members became members of staff, some became residents. Some were more off this planet than any resident I had yet to meet. Before the start of a musical performance the musical director would be dispensing generous doses of Rescue Remedy. On one occasion a particularly sensitive member of the choir picked up some negative energy surrounding the castle remains. Responding without hesitation we loyally trooped out and, facing what was left of this once sturdy bastion, we extended positive energy towards it with our voices; it must have worked as it is still standing today!
It must be said that however hippy and bizarre the choir would seem they provided for their members a supportive and caring environment away from the stresses and strains of everyday life. They also provided some very special moments for their singers and gigs could be anything from touring America and singing with the London Community Gospel Choir down to entertaining in retirement homes with wartime songs or Christmas carols. In actual fact it was sometimes the least likely venues that gave the greatest feel good factor.
The type of music the choir tackled was very varied, ranging from traditional European folk songs (sung in the language of their country of origin) to songs originating from the American slave tradition to ancient English pieces – in Latin! A favourite visiting choir master with all the choir members was Michael Harper. He would arrive for a weekend workshop and inspire us with his enthusiasm and charisma.

In addition to these musical endeavours were annual events such as Maggie's farm. Each year Maggie and Wilm would open a field at their farm near Ely for a weekend of camping and music.

All manner of individuals would turn up and entertainment would go on late into the night.

Another popular musical fund raiser was the talent competition held at the Ffolkes Arms. Anyone with a song to sing or a tune to play would spend hours rehearsing in preparation. The compere was a media student who came fully attired in tuxedo etc. and entered into his role as if he had been born into it. The drink flowed, applause was generous, the lights were low and the judges kind. The success of the event was due not just to the efforts of the musicians but also to the wide range of friends in Helen, Dave and their staff's circles. These people turned out to many events and I hope their generosity was rewarded by a good night's entertainment.

The beginning of summer was marked by another musical occasion known as Judy's garden party. Judy lived in a large vicarage in a remote leafy village. Most of the village was owned by Tom and Sally and a visit to this beautiful place was like a step back to a previous century. The vicarage had an enormous garden and during the garden party friends, staff and residents would come and share picnics, browse amongst the stalls and of course listen to those who had kindly agreed to sing and play music.
A nominal charge was made for entry to the garden party and this was donated to the Mill charity. Tom and Sally would also readily invite Millers to the Hall's magnificent gardens and woodland.

A regular event that must not miss a mention was the pantomimes and shows put on by the Gayton Incidental Theatre Society (otherwise known as GITS). Helen, Dave and sometimes staff belonged to this organisation. The pantomimes would be loyally attended by Millers who would be rewarded amply by hilarious performances. The highlight of these has to be Helen suspended by wires playing Tinkerbelle in a production of Peter Pan.

Christmas was yet another time marked memorably by music.

There was no escape or excuse from doing a turn at the Christmas party even if it was just the little green frog song. There was however one song during the evening that no one wanted to miss and that was Dave's. The tune was immaterial but somehow Dave managed to capture the essence of the residents in the lyrics of the song perfectly. I don't recall the verses, but one chorus sticks firmly in my mind. It goes like this;-

> *Colourful people leading colourful lives*
> *Telling the world where to go*
> *The system's all right when the system's not shite*
> *Don't tell me different I know*

It was never unusual to hear the words 'Oh Helen, you didn't?!'. Well sometimes I did! As my reader I will let you see some of my scattier moments!

Technology and I do not go together!
Mobile phones had just become the new 'thing' to have. As always the lazy technophobe doesn't find out how to work them. I head off to a council meeting, late, as timekeeping is something else I'm not good at. The large conference table is full so I sit on the row of chairs at the back of the room. Fiona, our business manager, who is very efficient and always on time gives me one of her looks to silently tell me I'm late. There are several important looking speakers lined up at the front of the room and an overhead projector and so the scene is set for the conference. While the speakers inform us of ideas and plans for the future for our vulnerable adults you can hear a pin drop until a phone starts to ring. I think to myself 'Oh, I say, fancy not turning your phone off'. Everyone looks around to see who the culprit is, including me as the ringing is close by. Suddenly I think 'Oh no' – it's coming from my bag on the floor! I take it out while the proceedings have come to a halt. I have removed it from my bag and by now it's very loud. I have no idea how to turn it off; I smile and apologise to the room full of people and quickly head towards Fiona at the other side of the room as I know she will be

able to turn it off. She takes it from me and instantly silences it –
I scurry back to my seat!

Mobile phone – oh no not again! Incident two.

I have had my phone a whole week now and I am enjoying using
it, periodically. We have a young woman staying who was on an
assessment with us from Hellesdon hospital. The lady in
question could be a 'colourful character' and at times difficult to
manage.

She was staying with us with the understanding that if she felt
unwell, anxious and needed to go back to the hospital I would
take her. This would hopefully make her feel safe and in control.
Well, she obviously didn't feel safe and presented herself at the
office door where I was writing up some notes. I looked up and
saw a picture you would associate with a horror film. She had
scratched down both sides of her face, which looked a real mess,
though the cuts were superficial. I cleaned her up and we set off
back to the hospital in Norwich. We chatted away and she now
appeared relaxed.
We were not far from the house when I could suddenly hear
voices. I said to the young girl "Can you hear voices?" She
looked at me and said yes to which I replied that I could too. We
continued on our journey and I could still hear voices. They
were distant and muffled. "I can still hear voices, can you?" I
asked. "Yes" she replied. I checked the radio but that was
switched off. I could faintly hear somebody calling my name,
"Helen......Helen". I pulled into the lay-by to investigate further
when I found my phone. I picked it up and could hear the voice
calling my name. I put it to my ear and said 'Hello'. "You've
left your phone turned on" – it was the Mill staff who had been
calling and shouting down the phone as they could hear me
talking and obviously knew that I would be running up quite a
phone bill! I look back on that journey and can't believe I kept
asking the young woman if she could hear voices. It was
probably the cause of her scratching her face in the first place;
she probably thought I was 'potty'!

We had so many adventures and as a consequence so many stories to tell. Things that might seem crazy, strange or ludicrous to others became normal for all at the Mill because these sorts of things happened daily. There are so many funny, strange and wonderful stories it would be impossible to write them all – here's a taster;

Gingivitis:

"Helen, Boots the chemist are on the phone". I thought to myself 'what do they want?'
"We have one of your residents here and she is refusing to leave the pharmacy. She has taken her teeth out and they are on the counter. She says she is not going anywhere until we give her some antibiotics. I have explained that they have to be prescribed by a doctor but she is not taking no for an answer." I asked the assistant to pass the phone to the resident and said very firmly – "Pick your teeth up, put them back in your mouth and get the next bus home. We will talk about this when you get here and sort it out with your doctor properly". She returned home on the next bus.
You have to admire her in some ways for fighting for what she thought she needed. Our intervention would be to ask for help appropriately.

Residents Rebel to Save the Chickens!

Although the Mill was a registered residential home most of us looked upon it as the 'communal good life'. We grew our own fresh vegetables and had our own chickens for eggs. We fattened a collection of chickens with the intention of having them killed at the local butchers and then eating them. However, this is where the residents rebelled. I called into the local butchers and booked a slot in the abattoir at the end of the week, ready for our hens to return home in neat plastic bags ready for the oven and freezer.
Banners were made and hung in the courtyard area and on the

front of the house. A cake was made for the visiting social workers and had the words 'save our chickens' iced on the top with fluffy hens. I did not want to keep the chickens and was determined that they would go. Thursday night we went home to our bungalow to return in the morning to take the hens to the butcher's. The morning arrived and Dave drew the curtains to start the day and was greeted with chickens running around the garden and our field. Chris, a member of staff, and residents had filled sacks and linen baskets with hens and driven up to our house and set them free! You can imagine trying to catch hens in a three acre field! The midnight chicken mission was talked about for many years after. The house buzzed with talk and laughter – what rebels!

Fund Raising Idea:

In the early days residents were given a very small amount of pocket money granted from the government. I was always looking for ways to raise a few quid to help support people living in the houses. We were paid fees for care and we funded as much as we could over and above what we were expected to in order to maximise everyone's quality of life. Money has never been a motivating factor for giving our residents choice, new experiences and educational opportunities. We were always happy to offer financial support. Fiona, our business manager, used to call us the Helen and Dave charity. Thankfully PALMS charity was formally set up in 1998 and this charity, named after Portland Street, Adrian Lodge and Mill House, now offers extra financial support for residents and ex residents.

Before PALMS we washed people's cars, had an occasional stall at the market, and had stalls at various friends' garden parties selling our unwanted goods. One of my 'brainwaves' in retrospect, was not such a good idea. We set off to the beach with a small trailer attached to the car. Seven of us picked armfuls of samphire and loaded it on to the trailer. I thought we could take it door to door to sell and raise some money towards a trip to France. We took our samphire back to the Mill and bagged it up before heading off to Grimston village to sell it. What great initiative, I thought. We soon sold out, although one lady did complain and say that it was full of cow samphire and not good to eat. Everyone really enjoyed themselves so we thought we would do it again soon. That was until I saw in the local paper that someone had been fined £450 for picking a trailer full of samphire with intent to sell. I couldn't believe it, I thought it was free for anyone to pick. I didn't realise you had to be licensed and have formal permission. We had often gone down to the marsh to collect a bag of samphire for tea. We all ooh'd and aah'd and discussed the what ifs and all agreed we had had a lucky escape.

The Television:

We arrived home from a week's holiday away with the boys. As the car came into the drive we were met by our Nigerian prince who was staying with us. He was clearly desperate to speak to us.

"I have done something really stupid and I'm so sorry" were his first words. I asked him what the problem was and he told me that he had stolen the television! "Why?" I asked. "Well," he replied, "I decided to go on a drug and drink binge and then kill myself, so I sold your television to get enough money to do it. I stole the television out of your sitting room, sold it, and went off to get drink and drugs. Anyway, I had a really good night and decided I didn't want to die, so I haven't killed myself but I have stolen your telly!" We thanked him for his honesty and said he could work the debt off and we would find him some paid work around the house. This was not an unusual thing for us to do. When people needed extra cash for a packet of fags or have an unforeseen expense we would be creative in finding some paid work. I think this helped keep some residents from taking things that didn't belong to them. We had very little in the way of theft and dishonesty.

WORSE THINGS HAPPEN AT SEA!

I look back and think 'Oh my God'!

It was a bright sunny day; just right for a picnic. Our little boat 'The Jolly Roger' was anchored at Burnham Overy harbour just waiting to take us on an adventure. The adventure was to motor around the creek and have fun. Six of us set off with Len as our captain in his blue sailor's cap. The water was shallow and providing we kept away from the sandbanks we were fine. As we all became more confident, Scolt Head Island seemed like a good destination and super location for our picnic and swim. We pulled up alongside the island and searched for a suitable anchor using an old wooden crate we filled with sand after securing the boat. We swam, laughed, ate and sunbathed. We talked to a group of people who had come to the island on the local ferry boat.

We decided to leave the island once we saw the ferry boat coming to collect its last passengers of the day. We hadn't thought about the tide coming in and the conditions changing. Rather quickly the shallow slim creek was filling up. We saw the ferry boat coming out in the distance, which was our cue to leave. We had had a fabulous time and hopped in the boat with Jake, who was only a baby, and headed for home. Lindsay insisted that she have a turn at being helmsman on the way back and reluctantly Len passed over the tiller. With our new captain at the helm it was only a short while before we were on a sandbank and stuck. Several attempts to restart the motor were to no avail as so much sand was now clogging the motor and we could only achieve a cough and a splutter. We were drifting with the tide. I was thinking of a plan of action when Len informed me that he couldn't swim – yes, wait for it – none of us had a life jacket. How irresponsible to say the least! I suggested that he hold onto the rope attached to the front of the boat and if the worst scenario happened he could hold onto it until he was rescued, as there were plenty of other boats about and ours would not sink. The others on board were all swimmers except, of course, my baby, Jake. But I knew that as a trained life guard and strong swimmer I could rescue him. The bank was not far away as we drifted down the creek.

Anyway, along comes the ferry boat and we all call for help. We are all laughing as the ferry boat comes alongside us and asks if we want a tow. The people who we had been talking to on Scolt Head are laughing. The captain of the ferry boat asked us to throw him our rope – the one Len is still holding on to! Our rope was just about a foot long and not nearly long enough to reach across and act as a tow rope. The captain looks at us with bemusement when we tell him it's our only rope, and soon has us attached with his substantial tow rope and tows us to shallow water near the shore. We get out and push the boat back to its anchorage. As we bend over to wash the mud from our legs we are approached by a man who has been watching the whole thing with his binoculars. He said "My wife dragged me out here this morning. I didn't want to come but I haven't laughed so much in a long time. If you give me your address I will send you some photos of the whole thing!".
He did, and they spent many years on the kitchen wall. We dined out on the story for years, it was so much fun. It never dawned on me that we were in danger! 'What ifs' don't bear thinking about!

Another group of residents came for a 'jolly' out at the seaside. It was one of those irresistible warm summer evenings. The sea was calling and I just had to go. I asked if anyone wanted to bring their swimming stuff and come for a swim or paddle. A small group came along and three of us walked a long way out to meet the sea. The water felt warm. We laughed and chatted away, not realizing that we had crossed a channel and this was filling up fast as the tide had turned and was coming in behind us. We turned to retreat back to shore. At first we had sand under our feet and the water was up to our knees. But soon the water was up to our shoulders and we had to swim across the channel. I felt we had to go. It didn't look that far and soon the shallow water the sea side of the channel would disappear and we would be in real trouble! I tried to be positive and said 'Oh isn't this fun, we'll soon be there'. Lorraine and Peter were competent but not what I'd call strong swimmers.

What a relief when we could feel our feet on the sand again. Both Lorraine and Peter continued to have anywhere between a smile and a look of confusion on their faces! Lorraine has since told me that she is extra careful at the beach now and really enjoys swimming in swimming pools – another lucky escape!

Lillian was a new member of staff and Powers, one of the residents, suggested a trip to Hunstanton because he wanted to try out his new life jacket as the following week Dave was taking him sailing. On arriving at Hunstanton the tide was a long way out. Some residents were happy to relax at the beach hut whilst the more adventurous people started the long walk out to the sea. Lillian suggested it was too far and that they should turn back. The group protested and carried on. Powers was soon floating around enjoying his new life jacket. The others had a swim and started to wander back. Before long they realized the tide was coming in behind them, unknown to them, one of the biggest of the year! They were now effectively on a sandbank. They had sea all around them and they were all now petrified. They continued to head towards the shore but the tide was now so high they had to swim. One very fit lad swam ahead, leaving the others. The tide took him a long way down the beach but he made it to the shore. Powers was scared but his new life jacket was keeping him afloat. Lillian had one of the girls on her back and was reassuring and calm. Someone on shore had luckily called the lifeboat which soon came and rescued them. The story was published in the local paper. Thankfully Lillian had spent much of her life as part of a circus where being strong and fit was essential. She had only been working for us for two weeks – what a start! We soon purchased a tide clock which hangs in the beach hut. In the twenty-five years we worked and lived at the Mill we lost nobody through suicide, which we were all very proud of. This may sound strange, but taking your own life is not an alien concept for people who have mental health problems. It's ironic that near death experiences could have happened while residents were out having fun.

We always had the best staff team I could dream of. Their dedication was immense and I loved working with them. They all had different, wonderful attributes and many of them are now close friends. I felt proud that these glorious people worked with me and Dave. They helped to make the Mill what it was and is.

They have their stories to tell too, some funny, some difficult.

Maureen, staff member;

The day I was the Devil!

Our home provided support to people in crisis who would benefit more from the home's environment than the Psychiatric Ward in the local hospital. On one occasion we had a chap in who was struggling with his mental health. His case manager had failed to mention that as part of his risk management plan he should not drink any alcohol or he could become quite violent. During an evening shift, when I was working alone, he returned from the local pub. Sitting opposite from him and a female resident in the kitchen I realised I had cause for concern when he started to display some psychotic symptoms. He had lots of tattoos on his arms, some of which were Gargoyles, he started to point at them and then at me. He had difficulty with his speech and was intimating that I was the devil and suggested that I had 666 tattooed on my forehead. He got quite distressed and would not be consoled or reassured that this was not the case. He then became more animated and got up to stand behind me. I was looking to the side so I could see his reflection in the glass panes of the kitchen doors, avoiding looking directly at him in case he thought I could read his thoughts. I could see that he was communicating with the female opposite me and was pointing at my head, and then running his hand across his throat as if to act out cutting it open. I was becoming more than a little nervous, my mind going at twenty to the dozen trying to think my way out of the situation, when he suddenly made his way to the top end of the kitchen to the large pot we kept the kitchen knives in! This was the point at which I thought it best if I got out of the way. I went to the office, (locked it) and called Dave who was always on call for emergencies. During the call I heard the chap coming after me. He tried the door and I shook from head to toe. Shortly afterwards Dave arrived, reassured me that I was right to leave the area as it was me the chap was preoccupied with and then went to deal with the situation. I went home.

A lot of responsibility:

One of our male residents became very unwell. He had suicidal thoughts and was struggling with 'voices'. He was taken to hospital, assessed and detained on the psychiatric ward. During one of the weekly ward rounds he was deemed fit enough to have some leave and so a visit to the Mill was arranged. We were told that he needed to be supervised whilst there and so I was keeping a close eye on his movements. He decided to go to the bathroom (a delicate balance between the right to some privacy and keeping someone safe came into play). I stayed close by but had to communicate briefly with another resident whilst he was in the bathroom. I turned my head for a moment at which point he disappeared. Within moments of his disappearance I alerted the staff but we really struggled to find where he had gone. We searched the house, the village, the fields, the derelict buildings in the area, alerted the hospital, police, but had no luck. Eventually, Helen and Dave decided, after the derelict buildings had been searched about half a dozen times, that they should search them again. They found him in a loft; there was no evidence of how he could have got up there. He was scared and confused and had heard commands from his 'voices' with suggestions that he was not safe in the house. They encouraged him to come down and he was returned to a safe environment. The realisation of how difficult it was to ensure this young man was kept safe really scared me.

Embarrassing moments:

I managed for a couple of years to avoid the inspector of our services mainly by giving the impressions that I lived there during his visits. He would turn up announced and I would sit on the sofa and watch TV. Unfortunately he eventually realised I was staff and so he met with me and another member of staff in the office to go through our systems etc. He asked me to answer some queries about medication and so, to placate him, I told him I would go and fetch the staff member who could be the most helpful to him. At the time I was wearing a sarong; it came down to my ankles and was wrapped around my waist twice and tied in a knot at the back. Unfortunately, just as I was going thought the office door the knot undid itself and my sarong dropped to the floor. I found myself standing there in my knickers with a cup of tea in one hand and the door handle still in the other. To add insult to injury my knickers were on inside out!

Then there was the night I was requested by my boss to ask a male resident (a biker) to stop masturbating at his bedroom window. This resident had recently informed me he had sexual dreams about me (he liked to shock) and when I went to his room and was invited in, I found him in bed. Whilst I stood in the doorway making my request he had one hand under the sheet! This situation seemed to keep him amused for some time.

There was the time when my boss, in her wisdom, encouraged me to join in with the tea dancing group. I got involved so as to encourage the residents to exercise and stick to their commitment once in the group. We had attended for weeks when two of the residents got married. They were having their reception/party afterwards in the Mill. Helen decided that we should 'perform' for the family and other guests who had gathered in the conservatory. We ended up dancing to Zorba the Greek. It was hilarious, there we were attempting to dance with our arms over each other's shoulders (everything bar the plate smashing) but none of us were very good. We ended up falling into people's laps who were sat very closely behind us, treading on old ladies toes etc. I could have done without that experience.

I worked for Helen and Dave for eleven years. Employment came after spending time with Helen on a playing field. I was watching a man playing with the kids in such a respectful and real way. The kids were enjoying the roundabout, swings etc., and joined in on a level they could relate to and appreciate. I expressed to Helen that I would love to be around people like him and that I felt my life was in a rut. She told me that he was a friend of hers; he turned out to be someone who had lived at the Mill and would come back from time to time for short stays. She invited me to her garden and after a Pimms and a chat with her and Dave I was invited to visit the Mill. My first impression of the place was that it was like a commune. I was unable to identify who lived there and who worked there (which I loved) and there was complete respect of each and all. I was asked if I would consider working there if a job ever came up. I was keen, to say the least. The next day Helen called me explaining that a post would be available in a couple of weeks; she offered me the job and I explained that whatever happened I would take her up on her offer and I did.

I can say, in all honesty, that until the day Helen and Dave announced their retirement I looked forward to going to work; every day was an adventure, sometimes good, sometimes bad or sad but the experiences could only serve to build character and make one humble. Here are some of the experiences most prominent in my mind.

Wonderful People:

Saxafraz:

A gap student from Australia spent one year with us, working alongside the staff team. She was full of sunshine, inside and out. She exuded enthusiasm which was infectious. She would busk in town, playing her guitar with residents who could also play and rather than worry about shoppers ignoring them, she would start singing about them as they passed by which invariably resulted in them smiling at least. The same girl was mad about a group called the Waifs (an Australian band). She would play their CDs in the Mill and lots of residents came to enjoy the music. She discovered the band were to play in London which resulted in staff and residents going to the gig. The first night they went the people who live at the Mill took with them a large handmade card full of messages of appreciation and good wishes and gave it to the Waifs. Such a good time was had that they went a second time (two nights later) which is when the Waifs handed out flowers to them and expressed their appreciation for their enthusiasm. Later in the year a large parcel come to the Mill addressed to the residents; it was from the Waifs. They had sent the lead singers a guitar, signed by the band, with the offer of a music workshop the next time they were in England.

Our wonderful friends played a big part in our life at the Mill. They were always on hand if needed and we appreciated their kindness and support. Here is an offering from Linda K, my good friend and someone with whom I have worked for a number of years. I believe her account sets the scene in a very honest manner to give you a flavor of her thoughts of Community Support Homes;

'Memories of Mill House, Gayton and Dave & Helen of course':

I first met Dave and Helen in the spring/summer of 1988 a few months after I lost my eldest son. It was a very difficult time for me but I was introduced to them at one of their summer parties. I didn't want to go home because I was having such a good time. However, the people I went with did want to go, so I was given the offer of staying the night, which was very hospitable. Unfortunately they seemed to have some difficulty finding sufficient bedding for everybody and I finished up on the sofa with a bright yellow candlewick bedspread which had been retrieved from the dirty washing. So I slept in my clothes with my curly perm stuck to one side and being serenaded and/or propositioned by another guest (a Social Worker) for most of the evening as he was busy strumming away on his guitar and refusing to go to bed. I woke up in the morning with a crick in my neck, my hair looking most peculiar and lots of yellow fluffy bits stuck to my beautiful black dress. Now this should have warned me that while Dave and Helen are extremely inclusive and open and very willing to provide hospitality to people, they are not all that nurturing and caring when it comes to looking after the finer things in life. You are expected to be self-resourcing in this respect. Despite their very supportive ways, occasionally their approach left something to be desired. They are truly caring people and, as lots of us who know them as friends have found, they have given incredible support and love over the years. We have quite unashamedly leaned on them to give us the kind of background of inclusiveness and unconditional regard that many of us have not managed to achieve in our own lives, or with our own families. The first evening proved to be the start of an association that has gone on for the last twenty years, and Dave and Helen have been the most amazing friends imaginable. Having said all that, you have to put up with an awful lot of insults.

Not that I didn't give as good as I got; quite a lot of teasing and general winding up. Everything they do is mostly done on their terms and you are very welcome to join in but don't expect to change their minds; it is not a democracy.

In the early days of running the Mill they had hardly any staff and fairly quickly after meeting them they decided to recruit me as I had some residential experience when I worked for Break even though I was a Probation Officer at the time. I was asked to take over the Mill while they went on holiday. Now this was always problematic because somehow they never seemed to quite brief you properly. All the occasions are somewhat muddled up in my mind, but I'll pick out the highlights, or in some people's estimations, the low lights, of my experiences of managing the Mill in Dave and Helen's absence. They ran the Mill on a very family based principal, and were Mum and Dad. The minute Mum and Dad went away, predictably, all the siblings started to play up badly. Being left in charge overnight by one's self was a bit of a daunting prospect, and one evening in particular sticks out in my memory.

Residents were competing for my attention, they were fighting with each other, and were generally causing mayhem so I decided that the best plan was to remove myself from the situation so that they couldn't act up for my benefit any more. Having said that, I was extremely worried and finding it very difficult to cope with the behaviour that was being thrown at me so I finished up skulking in the office. I secretly telephoned Dave Butterworth, a fellow Probation Officer, trying to get some support for my isolation and the chaos that I could hear rising in the house next door. In the end I decided well, I'll take myself to bed, so off I went. It's the coldest bedroom you have ever been in your life, I have no idea where that temperature came from. Anyway, I am lying in bed, shivering slightly and waiting, and sure enough, bang-bang-bang-bang-bang-bang, I hear people coming up the stairs bang-bang-bang along the corridor. There were two doors between Dave and Helen's bedroom and the house, crash there's one fire door and bang-bang-bang on the other one. "Come quick, somebody's broken a window" – so down I have to go to deal with the chaos. Somebody had broken a window, claiming they had done it while they were asleep, two people were arguing over the television etc. etc. etc. I did manage to quieten them down in the end but I don't think I got any sleep that night!

Chaos threatened to break out when I was casually informed before I started one sojourn at the Mill that Helen's uncle might be coming to lay the living room carpet. Well if you had any idea about how much use that living room got and what a nightmare it would have been if I had to move everything to fit the carpet then you can understand I was panicking slightly. Never mind, they weren't quite sure what was happening, and in the end, thankfully, he didn't turn up. On another occasion something dodgy happened with the horrible little electric toilet upstairs that nobody was allowed to put tampons or condoms down, because it all had to be mashed up blah blah. Anyway I had to call the plumber, who was a fairly unpleasant young man but the one benefit of it was that Sally the dog managed to grab hold of his ankle and all I could see was him standing in the utility room desperately shaking his leg trying to get the dog off. That was the only time we liked that dog. Another of the problems working at the Mill was when taking phone calls from referring professionals. I remember one particular occasion, somebody phoned up to ask for the criteria for taking people into the Mill, which left me in some confusion because I was well aware that the main criteria was, would Helen like the person being referred or not? It wouldn't matter how disastrous or chaotic the person had been, providing Helen liked them and she could see a positive placement for them in the house. So I had to cobble something up and tell terrible lies about, I don't know, behaviour modelling, family structure and whatever else; anyhow I got by. What I did learn about people with mental health problems is that they can be more accepting and non judgemental than some people in what we would call normal society. There was never a day when you went into the kitchen at the Mill and weren't offered coffee or a cigarette or to sit down or a chat with somebody there who may not even know you from Adam, and you did wonder at that time who was the 'mad' one. It was also impossible to tell who was a resident, who was a friend, who was a worker and who were the owners. We all seemed to operate on more or less the same level of friendship and connection and nobody was introduced as anything; we didn't have labels.

All social occasions and most of family life took place in and around the Mill with the residents integrating into whatever was going on, as indeed did friends. Some of the highlights were of course the Christmas pantomimes. I have to say that some of them were the most extremely ridiculous situations you can imagine. I remember one particular young man, a beautiful large black guy called Julian, playing baby Jesus wrapped in a large white towel and nothing else. I was cast as the Angel Gabriel in this particular production, which involved me wearing a lovely shiny top and bit of a halo and probably a short skirt or shorts, because we did seem to show a lot of leg and fishnet tights etc. in those days, and I had to enter the scene on a bicycle. Not being the best person on two wheels, I entered screaming as the whole thing seemed to be horribly out of control. I slid across the room and crashed into the chair on the opposite side, causing a great deal of hilarity; this has probably not been forgotten to this day.

One of the drawbacks of this particular production was that I had to do dirty dancing with Dave Butterworth. Now, not only is that quite a dreadful thing to imagine, he didn't seem to have any flexibility in his hips, so while he seemed to be able to pogo up and down, sexually moving his hips from one side to the other didn't seem to be in his repertoire. Also he has a very hairy chest.

Some of the characters at the Mill were actually larger than life. One particular resident, we'll call MC was a really large scary, dominating looking man who sounded very clever. He could make himself sound cynical and sarcastic and very knowing. Unfortunately he treated himself to a tiny ridge tent. He was attempting to put this up in the garden while I was on duty at the Mill one day, only he hadn't quite mastered the method of putting up a tent. He put the inner liner up and hung it from the poles, which was quite successful; a nice bright posh liner. He then thought he'd climb in it to see exactly how it felt. Unfortunately it seemed to be slightly smaller than MC himself but he eased himself into it as I came down the garden to see how he was getting on and said "How are you doing, MC?", whereupon there was some strange gyrating like a large overgrown pupa which revealed that the liner had in fact entirely engulfed his body and was sticking to it. His head being shoved up the end with no exit, he was in some distress about how he was going to get out but was busy trying to tell me that all was fine. It was very fortunate that his vision was obscured and I managed to stifle my uproarious hysterical giggling so that I didn't offend him completely. We negotiated for a while but in the end we decided that the only thing that could be done was for me to take the poles down and peel the liner off him so that he could be in the fresh air once more. I'm not sure what happened to that tent but I do hear tell that in another circumstance when he was camping, he decided he couldn't deal with the tent at all and just knocked it down!

Helen's ability to motivate the residents and force them all to live by her mantra of fresh air and exercise was admirable. I remember on one occasion there had been a lot of snow and she was determined that they were going to go out and 'enjoy' the environment. She spent about twenty minutes perambulating the house, geeing everybody up, bullying, shouting, cajoling and otherwise managing to get at least the mini bus full of people. And off they went to snowball. Inevitably, half of them fell over hurting themselves, hurt each other, slid down the hill without being able to control themselves and generally gave Helen a great deal of amusement. Then she brought them all home again. Fresh air and exercise had been achieved by all!

What was most striking about the experience for residents being at the Mill was to be accepted for exactly who they were and not be judged. I remember one resident, Mark, a very clever lad who really could wind people up and play the system, who hadn't been there very long when he managed to drop a whole pile of dinner plates and break every one, and he said to me that he got the most remarkable reaction! Helen had just said 'oh never mind, we've got some more, clear that up, there's some more in the cupboard,' and having expected to be bawled out and generally made to feel completely and utterly useless, he was gobstruck at this different approach, and recognised that he was hooked on the place for ever after.

Helen and Dave extend this understanding to all of their eccentric friends too. I certainly have misbehaved quite badly at times in the past, and while they may not have necessarily approved of what I have been doing they have never judged me or blanked me for any reason whatsoever. They are loyal, in fact you can say their loyalty is stronger in adversity than at any other time, for which I have been heartily grateful over the years, and hope they feel that I return an equal strength of regard and loyalty.

There was always something going on at the Mill – somebody was always taking the mickey out of somebody or playing a prank, and we all used to join in. When Helen brought one of her babies back from the hospital we erected the mast of the sailing dinghy that happened to be in the yard and draped across the whole parking space a line of nappies, which were artificially soiled with Branston Pickle, just to make her feel at home.

I once took over the Mill in the wake of a house holiday in France during which one resident had decided to stay behind to visit family. Unfortunately he hadn't got sufficient Methadone with him so on their return one of the carer support workers was trying to get a prescription sent out to him in France. This we weren't able to manage because it wouldn't be honoured in a pharmacy over there. The next plan was to pack a bottle of Methadone in a parcel to send to him. However, we checked this out with Customs and that wasn't permissible either. So when the gentleman phoned up we were unable to provide him with any means of getting his Methadone, which you can imagine did cause a fair amount of stress. After a couple of days of highly charged calls trying to sort this problem out it was decided that the only way round this was to come home before his supply ran out. Unfortunately he also had no money either. I pointed out there was little I could do to help him at this stage, and he needed to get himself to a ferry port in which case I would then try and get him sufficient funds to get a ferry home. There then followed a series of reverse charge phone calls from all across France of various degrees of irritation on his part and mine. At one point I snapped "So what do you want now?". Eventually he made it to Calais and I had to phone Dave and Helen who were away on holiday and get their holiday home owners to attract their attention in order to get some kind of a credit card off them in order to get the gentleman home. He got home safely, but I don't think he ever forgave me and seemed to hold me entirely responsible for his inability to stay in France and receive his medication.

Even when not at the Mill I would bump into the residents in and around Kings Lynn and elsewhere, and on one particular occasion I was walking through the town centre when, unusually, there was a gentleman under a gazebo in a complete evening suit with dickie bow singing opera to a beat box that he had beside him. During the break in his performance I noticed one of the Mill residents advancing upon him, pulling her lip back with her forefinger in order to reveal to him her gingivitis that she felt everybody should be informed about, and I must admit that at that point I did a quick whiz round the back of the gazebo and down an alley in order not to be drawn in to this particular conversation.

I have found it difficult to recall some of the details of the more traumatic events at the Mill, probably to protect my own mental health, but the worst night at the Mill was when there was a resident there called Marge who was a huge Goth, completely out of control really. She used to play her music at the top of its volume which caused her to be attacked verbally by a fellow resident, Debbie, who shouted and banged doors. In the meantime I was in the office which was in between their two bedrooms with this poor guy Kris who had his head in his hands, saying "if I die the whole world dies, therefore I can't commit suicide". In the meantime I could hear the banging and the crashing and the escalation of the shouting going on outside the door which considerably racked up my anxiety as you can imagine. What really got through to me from Kris's conversation was that I really understood how difficult it is to live life when you don't even know whether your thoughts are your own, and your whole way of living and decisions about behaviour is dependent on the level and the ferocity and the control of the voices inside your head. I learnt a lot about mental health that night. I also learnt a lot about the difficulties of trying to manage a lot of very cross, demanding, attention-seeking and out of control people, with common sense, care and compassion, and for me I think retreating to the office in those circumstances was probably the safest option.

Meeting Dave and Helen, living and working alongside them and trying to understand and relate to people's mental health problems gave me some of the most profoundly positive experiences in my life. I've moved on to establish a good friendship circle and gained a better understanding of the importance of a sense of belonging, tolerance, loyalty and support in everybody's lives. I have been a beneficiary of the values that Dave and Helen hold and practice, despite the fact they are monstrous people and complete control freaks who like everything their own way!! But they are warm, very funny, committed to the well being of others, have great perception of how people work, are completely inclusive and altogether have provided me and, I suspect, all the people they have cared for through the Mill House and Community Support Homes with a solid sense of belonging and a unique experience of respect and care. All this has contributed to me being able to move on, and it has given the vast majority of people they have worked with exactly the same. But most of all we feel loved and we love you too. Thank you.

Dave Butterworth – otherwise known as D.B., a dear friend who was always ready to help regardless of the request. For example, one night I rang him and Dave and asked them to come home from their quiet drink at the local because I was in labour and was having contractions every ten minutes (the residents were very excited). On their return we had a quick coffee and D.B. returned to his home offering his help and support if we needed it. At 4am we asked D.B. to return to look after the Mill as I was in the last stages of labour. He was soon back. Handing over necessary information was not straightforward, as each time I had a contraction D.B. sang at very fast speed a nursery rhyme to keep me distracted until the pain subsided. Jake was born at 5am at the local hospital and we were soon home.
Another request was "Can you come on holiday with us?"

D.B. in France:

It all began with an innocent enough question sometime in the late 1980's... What are you doing for 2 weeks in July? Do you think you could help with a holiday for the Millers to the South of France? Well, Dave and Helen are old and good friends and I'm a frequent visitor to The Mill and know the residents, so I book a couple of weeks off and hey let's go for it.

Now The Mill is like an extended family with friends and relatives dropping in – that's friends and relatives of the Millers and of Dave and Helen, so it's all very relaxed (most of the time). I was a bit concerned that this relaxation might get carried over to the organisation. The plan was to use two vehicles, a newish Toyota minibus and an oldish but large Citroen 7 seater estate, with two drivers per vehicle. We were to head off early from Gayton to Dover and then down via Lyon to Hyeres where we'd all camp. Helen had ducked out of the drive down, claiming car sickness, and was flying to Marseilles, Dave was to drive the Toyota and I was to drive the Citroen. The Citroen, as I mentioned, is oldish, well to be exact rather dilapidated, so I am pleased to learn that it has been fully serviced and checked before we go.

Early in the morning, around 4.00am if I remember correctly, we are all loaded and head off, with Dave in the lead from Gayton for the three to four hours' drive to Dover. All goes well for the first 4000 yards or so, then the Citroen, which has lots of lights on the dashboard, has a huge one lit up in red: "STOP". This is before mobile phones, and we haven't got a radio. Dave has disappeared ahead, the village garage is closed, the brakes, steering and everything else seem to work and I hope he notices that we are not behind him and waits for me to catch up. We meet up at the big roundabout in Kings Lynn where Dave tells me there was a bit of a problem with the hydraulics – for those not acquainted with earlier Citroens, everything from the lift up suspension to the brakes and steering all rely on the hydraulics! We top up, the light goes out, the can goes in a safe place and we eventually arrive in Dover.

One of the things about the Millers and others with mental health problems is that they have a variety of difficulties, and cross channel ferries have bars that open when you're on them. What we discover on starting off on the motorway from Calais are three things. One of my charges is desperate for a pee; we have not devised any method of communicating with the others vehicle; Dave is desperate to put some miles between us and Calais. A fairly rudimentary but effective system of flashed lights, three flashes on the indicator indicates that a stop is required. First pee stop about five miles from Calais! A good sign, but French motorway cafes do good coffee so I'm okay.

Many seemingly uneventful hours later, we're looking for somewhere to pitch the tents for the night. We don't really want to go through Lyon as it's getting late and there don't seem to be too many camp sites around. So, sometime around 10pm we pull off having found a site. By then it's late, we've been travelling for something like 16 hours and, frankly, we're knackered. The weather is good, so we decided to erect the outer of a frame tent and all crawl into it for the night. Bliss! Germans have a reputation for efficient organisation which seems to extend to camping trips. We arrive late and the rest of the site is peacefully asleep so no one has witnessed the 18 or so disappearing inside one frame tent, about 12ft x 12ft. Our neighbour's face, a German gentleman, was a picture as what seems like a bus load emerges the next morning from a tent built for 4 – 6.

Next mistake: Rush hour in Lyon is horrendous.

By now it is very hot. We finally arrive in Hyeres. The site is typically "South of France"; dusty, bamboo, ditches, but close to the beach.

Remember Helen? She is flying in to Marseilles. By which I mean I am envious of her comfortable journey! While Dave and the others put up the tents, I head off to Marseilles airport. This is of course pre satnav as well as pre mobile phone. Out map is not brilliant, but finding the airport can't be difficult, can it? There are signs for Aerospatiale which take us through Marseilles. It's rush hour. Police cars with sirens ignore the one way streets and head straight at you. It turns out Aerospatiale is not the airport. Eventually we find the airport, and Helen. On arrival back at camp I am so exhausted I slither down the side of the car into a heap on the ground.

A little later all is well again, we get some sleep and look forward to the following day. The guy who had a bit too much lager on the ferry heads off with a friend to explore the village a couple of miles away. That's fine, until they don't turn up for supper. Search party, all the bars, no sign – up and down the streets, no sign. Much later just as we're about to visit the local Police, these two turn up having discovered the joys of French bars. The next morning they discovered the joy of cleaning out their tent after adverse reactions to the drink.

What goes with a camp site that is dry and hot with ditches around it? 'Mossies' of course, which happily focussed their attention on one young woman, who in turn happily scratched and scratched and scratched against all our efforts to persuade her otherwise, until her legs looked like she had smallpox!

The rest of the time there was brilliant, all the residents and 'staff' had a great time and then the time came to leave.

We're all packed. The cars are loaded to the gunnels. The roof racks are full of bags. Dave did promise me that the Citroen had been fully checked and serviced before we left UK, didn't he? The most important driver mirror in France is the one on the left hand side of the car. The mirror on the Citroen is held on by insulation tape. It's exceedingly hot as we leave on the motorway, heading north. And what happens to insulation tape when it's hot? As we're on the motorway, the mirror detaches itself and hangs banging on the side of the car by the wire that operates the remote control adjuster. Great! Can you just hang out of the window please and hold the mirror in place until we get to some place we can fix it? Thanks

Our overnight stop on the way back is better paced than on the way down. Same procedure in reverse, one frame tent outer, everyone in for the night.

Unfortunately the ground has a slope and the first person in and to sleep is positioned so they'll naturally roll down the slope when they move in their sleep. We start off evenly spaced; next morning 50% of the floor space is vacant and we're in a heap against one side of the tent. We discover that someone has packed their passport in their bag, which is on the roof of the car, with the load secured and covered by tarpaulins. We're delayed a wee bit by not having a clue which bag it's in, or in *which car. He can't remember. Ah well.*

The last leg involves a journey around the Paris ringroad. Dave's in the lead vehicle, the Toyota minibus. He's got the map, but sadly no one in his vehicle can read it. I'm practically tail gaiting him so we don't get split up. Dave seems to be looking at the map – has he spotted that tipper truck in front breaking? Just in time the Toyota's nose goes hard down, the back lifts up and we narrowly miss accident number 5691 on the ringroad.

Well, Helen is flying back to the UK in comfort. But I would not have missed this trip for the world. What a great bunch of people. All difficulties overcome. All nicely tanned. All happy, with lots of stories to tell.

CHAPTER FIFTEEN

Another staff member was Bev who laughed like a drain, was sometimes clumsy in her approach, would go through a brick wall to fight for people's rights and had an infectious personality. Singing, dancing, cooking and acting are just some of her talents and she became Outreach Manager extraordinaire!

Her story:-

If Oscars were being given out my acceptance speech would be:

'I'd like to thank my dad for my wit and humour, for on so many occasions this saved me. Many times I have thought 'My God, I'm only a barmaid' and have been at a loss as to what to say or do when people have been experiencing their darkest moments. If lost for words I have danced to Kylie Minogue and other pop tunes to try and defuse a situation I have found myself in. I have laughed, cried and often felt 'Wow, I'm actually being paid for having so much fun'.

Driving the minibus taught me skills I never imagined I possessed. Navigation and emergency stops were my forte. For example, when driving on the M25 and one of my passengers decided to flash their boobs to a bloke in the next lane, I thought it best to slow down. I have also written off the works car, ending up in a ditch.

In my time I have made people play football and join in exercise classes when they have overdosed on paracetamol or broken their arm.

Still, I was told that I was fantastic fun and a good team player! I don't think I will ever meet such an amazing group of people as those in the Homes, whom I still look on as my extended family.

When working on those long overnights I would tell residents that I would make breakfast the next morning, thinking that the thought of my culinary skills would stop them from waking me up at night. I was so naïve, but in a way it helped me do the job. Tuesday morning staff meeting was the highlight of the week and I don't think I've ever laughed so much. I have been truly spoilt for the rest of my career, but I will not accept anything less from jobs, employers and work colleagues. As Helen always used to say, 'the proof is in the pudding', and I've tasted the best pudding ever!

Bev is the outreach manager, which means that she supports residents in their own home. It is a step from residential care, as staff will assist and support for an hour a day. For a time she worked as manager of Adrian Lodge, one of our sister houses. She has more tales to tell;

Training day:

We were told that after lunch we would be doing some role play. Yippee! I love a bit of role play; must be the actor in me!
The training guy called me from the room into the corridor to give me instructions.
He said, "one of your residents has gone to a police station to confess a murder he committed in 1989",
"Yes....." I said, waiting with baited breath for more instructions.
He repeated "One of your residents has gone to the police station to confess to a murder in 1989."
"Ye-es....." I repeated, wondering if I was getting the idea right.
"No! This is for real. One of your residents actually has gone to the police station to confess a murder and you need to get there now!"
"Flippin' heck" I shrieked, ran and grabbed my coat and left!
It later turned out that Scotland Yard had indeed been involved – but the murder was a delusion of a mentally ill man.

Mad or Bad:

After collecting a resident from the psychiatric ward after consultants and doctors assured me that there was nothing wrong with this person mentally and they would not be keeping him any longer I put him in my car and started to drive him home. A few seconds later he grabbed my face and hair with a look on his face that I will never forget. I slammed on the brakes and jumped out of my car, holding up the traffic. The police were called and he was escorted to the police station. The police informed me that they could not press charges because he was assessed for mental health issues and they thought it was a matter for the hospital, but they didn't agree and said it was a matter for the police! He was then sent home to our care and a couple of days later slit his throat, which he survived, and I knew that we couldn't ever have him back. I was scared, my staff were scared and I lost my trust in the 'system's' ability to decide who was mad or just plain bad.

Ann driving:

There is a huge field where we used to go camping with the residents. The whole event was called 'Maggie's Farm' and we would all have so much fun there. Sometimes the residents would have a go at driving around the field. I asked Ann, a resident, what she had been up to. "I had a driving lesson! Louise let me have a go at driving the car; it was great!" "Then Louise got stuck in the toilets". "What did you do"? I asked, "Oh, just sat on the floor and waited for her".
For someone who is deemed extremely mentally unwell by the professionals a bit of normality is all they need and deserve!

Judy – Highly qualified in mental health and the nursing profession, she has integrity, dignity, and respect for all and never does she compromise her beliefs, regardless of any situation. At our leaving party Judy and her husband Robin performed a song that Judy had written. I know this performance took Judy out of her comfort zone; we were so grateful for her kindness.

Her story follows;

When Helen and Dave retired I tried to summarize in the song below their achievements and dedication in providing services for the mentally ill.

I have worked in psychiatry since 1974 in various places, both in Norfolk and beyond. When I came across 'The Mill' and was given a job there, I found it had one of the best philosophies of enabling, respecting and encouraging people to have a positive outlook, to foster new beginnings, to have a chance to be treated as an individual. People believed in Dave and Helen and had faith in them as people. This was my experience and it was my favourite working place.

Helen and Dave had a great vision of how to develop a service to meet needs as they arose. They took huge risks both with people and properties. Their boundless energy and creativity in providing support and encouragement was unceasing. They were always looking at new ways to approach problems and encouraging others to do the same.

Their consistent approach of including people in the community and everyday life not only benefited the people but educated others in mental health issues and attempted to bridge the gap between 'them' and 'us' which unfortunately remains a huge issue in our society.

Being large providers in mental health care in West Norfolk, their reputation spans over a wide area. They never forgot anyone who had used their service and would constantly be on call for a wide range of people. They were and still are a 'rock' to a lot of people.

As employers they used the same approach to bring out the best in their staff, had belief in them and allowed and encouraged them to be creative and to take calculated risks. As an employee, I always felt very safe and supported, which enabled me to retain my enthusiasm, energy and positivity; I was also allowed to be argumentative! (Much appreciated). I will always be very grateful for the way they created jobs to fit round my personal life and supported me totally; we had great times with lots of laughs and fun, but it was great in the bad times too.

It was a unique service allowing individuality, embracing all aspects of life and helping people to contribute and find their own strengths and potentials by providing such safe and unique environments. I don't think there will be another service quite like it, which is a real shame, but for the many who benefitted from it, Community Support Homes will remain a great part of their lives.

'THANK YOU FROM ALL' by Judy.

24 years ago
Helen and Dave 'the pair'
Bought a house called the Mill
And it stands right there
(Chorus)
Oh what a pair
And how did they care

Beds were offered to all
The small the big and the tall
Were knocking on the door
No more room on the floor
(Chorus)

Soon the word got out
What the Mill was about
More hands required
And Portland Street acquired
(Chorus)

Smiles tears and fears
Passed away the tears
Working day and night
Keeping everyone bright
(Chorus)

All the beds again taken
Some people being forsaken
A pub went up for grabs
And Adrian Lodge was nabbed
(Chorus)

24 hours a day
'The pair' got so old
He went very grey
They decided it must be sold
(Chorus)

What a loss to the people
The small the big and the tall
O how you'll be missed
But you're always top of our list
(Chorus)

A great big thank you from all
The small the big and the tall
Good luck in all you do
To a very deserved two
(Chorus)

(As sung by Judy and Robin at Helen and Dave's retirement party 15th September 2007)

Mary – Oh, how I wish we'd found you earlier!

I was 14. An age when we tend to think that adults know us more than we know ourselves, that they can see around corners, through doors, into our souls, and know when we are naughty, lying and deluding ourselves.

Our class were taking part in a careers' advice session. I now know this was wrongly labelled and should have been called a 'confidence destruction session' Our 'teacher' asked a few random pupils what they would like to be when they left school and when they answered, proceeded to tell them why they would be useless in their chosen field.
Nervous tittering came from the pupils who were not singled out. I was alarmed (and disturbed from my window gazing/daydreaming) when it was my turn to be humiliated.
When asked I answered that I would like to help people. "Help people! You can't even help yourself!" he exclaimed.

It wasn't until 35 years had passed by that I realised the importance of his words. Only when I asked Helen and Dave if they had any cleaning work available and they insisted that I was capable of much more and had a lot to offer did I realise that I had limited myself.
I worked for Helen and Dave as a support worker and gained so much from the experience; confidence, fulfilment and fun.

The point of this story is that Helen and Dave constantly showed this belief, that people are capable of so much more than they realise, to everyone, residents and staff alike. This is why they have helped countless people back to mental health, fulfilling happiness and self belief. Once learned, this belief can be passed on daily by staff to anyone who mistakenly believes they have nothing of value to offer society.

Angie – full of enthusiasm with an infectious drive for life:

I sat down to write an account of what my working life at the Mill gave me. I was surprised how emotional I felt and what a remarkable journey I had been on. I started with words that came into my head which reminded me of my experiences. I never did manage to put this into a story, but here are my words – which say it all!

Joy, lights, bonfire, busy, freedom, creativity, adventures, magic moments, the dogs – Megan, Holly, Lucy, Sally and Mo, laundry, family, children, warmth, happy, relaxed, gardening, meals, house chores, jumble, car boots, walks, the Dales, markets, swing chair, sunbathing, corners, fireside, people always popping in, plays, pantomimes, party, celebrations, spontaneity, sunshine, water fights, Steve Redgrave 5 x gold medallist, laughter, Tottenham, Derby County, Norwich City, education, alarm clock, Spring, safety, sweet wrappers, camping, policeman, European Cup Final, Man U 3 - 2 Bayern Munich, fliers, Dave's song lyrics, grow up, confidence, kitchen table, coffee, tea, cooking, weddings, comfort, support, Christmas, Birthdays, bets on the Grand National, sweepstakes, relaxed.
The opportunity to live, belong and be accepted and enhance everybody's life chances.

Fiona's Story;

I enjoyed living in the flat at Portland Street and my son, Ian, did too. He was given a picture of a house and asked to draw the people in his family in the windows. He drew 10 people. We are a very small family so I asked him who all the people were, and he started listing all the residents. We were going to the pictures one afternoon during the school holidays. As we walked out of the front door and closed it he asked where the people were. I said that they didn't want to come to this film. He was most put out and said he would be lonely. Clearly his mother was not sufficient company for him!

Ian enjoyed the various characters in the house and called them 'the people'. He found a strip of raffle tickets one day when he was about five years old and than went over to the flat and got a variety of items; a small Kit Kat, a car and various other toys. He laid them in the middle of the sitting room and after tea when everyone was sat in the sitting room he gave out all the tickets and made people throw the tickets at the 'prizes' in the middle of the room, and when their ticket touched a prize he declared they had one and gave them the prize.

In the mid 1990's we had to start recording the temperature of food that we were serving. Anne was putting the probe into the sausages in the toad in the hole she had taken out of the oven prior to serving it. Eric walked downstairs and watched her for a minute or two and then asked 'What are you doing?' She said 'Taking the temperature of the sausages'. He said 'Why, sick are they?'

When Jan came to live at Portland Street she had spent two years in the David Rice hospital and was very anxious and upset about moving. Jan had been sexually abused during her very troubled childhood. At thirteen, to get away from the abuse she went to live with her elder sister. This was not an easy move as her sister had an illegitimate mixed race child and was struggling with her own difficulties. Jan had overdosed and cut her arms on more than 80 occasions, sometimes quite severely. She woke me about 4 times a week in the middle of the night, crying, suicidal, wanting to return to her flat in Norwich. Gradually she calmed down and learnt to talk about her fears and anxieties during the day, and eventually we got her to see a psychologist who gained her trust and did eye movement and desensitisation with her which was like a miracle cure. She has since married, had a child and she and her husband run a successful business in Norwich. The whole family are a delight and I do not cease being amazed at the transformation.

Jenny came to live at Portland Street before she went on Clozapine medication and was not really stable enough to move out of hospital, but the system wanted her out. When I went to collect her the staff said they had not bothered packing much for her as she would not be likely to stay very long... They were right! She did not last the day. One of the many things she did to demonstrate her lack of stability was to go out into the road and lie down. It was not safe to leave her unattended as there were no waking night staff we had no choice but to take her back to hospital. Some months later when she had been stabilised on Clozapine she returned to Portland Street and spent several years there before moving to a rehab house and eventually sharing a flat where she still lives successfully.

Mark had severe auditory hallucinations and spent many hours talking to himself and answering, sometimes very noisily. On one occasion he was in his room, shouting to himself. Another resident lived in the next but one room and went out into the corridor and shouted to him to ask him to be quiet. He replied 'it's not me', which to him it probably wasn't, as it was his voices which were not him.

Ian lived with his mum Fiona, one of our managers at one of our sister houses. He was a small toddler when they moved into the flat integrated into the main house. Like most family houses there were different characters with their own type of behaviour. This household could be described as very eccentric at times, in the funniest of ways...

A Child's Viewpoint

For me, growing up in and around Portland Street and the other Homes was just normal. Obviously, I now know that most of the houses were anything but normal, in some of the funniest ways. A lot of the residents had their unusual habits which I thought were just bizarre or just plain funny. For example, at every shared meal time, Ray, one of the residents, would always sneeze because he'd put so much pepper on his food, then my mum would always talk to him about putting too much pepper on his food then the next meal time he'd do it all again.
When I was really young I would always tell the same joke to

*Ray every meal time without fail; 'Knock Knock.' 'Who's there?'
'Fish.' 'Fish who?' 'Bless you!' That was the joke I told every
meal time; I'm sure my mother loved that one. Then there was
Eric, he never said a lot but whenever he walked the dog he only
ever went to the end of the road and turned back. I remember
once, I thought the dog was really fat and to be honest she was,
so I decided to go with Eric and walked all round the park just to
try and get the dog thin. Being so young I expected all the fat to
come off in one walk but the dog nearly collapsed when we got
back. As I grew up I saw Eric quite often in Sainsbury's, because
they had escalators and every day he would enjoy riding them.
It would always make me smile when I saw him riding them.
Occasionally he would press the red button which stopped the
escalator in its tracks, with customers looking confused. Eric
always wore the same expression, never giving anything away.*

*I became quite attached to some of the residents. AK was one
person I remember well. She was really good at drawing and at
school I loved drawing so we would quite often sit in the
residents' sitting room and just draw whatever toys I could find. I
remember when my mum and I used to meet with AK after she'd
moved on into the community. We used to go to Downey's Cafe
and have a cream cake. It was always nice to see her.*

*Janine is another resident that I still see and get on very well
with. I think she is one of the big success stories. I was a page
boy at her wedding and she now owns her own business with her
husband. They have a beautiful little boy called Harry to whom I
am godfather.*

*My mum has always worked for the charity P.A.L.M.S which was
founded to help support the homes and residents past and
present. My mum completed the London Marathon a number of
years ago and after travelling down with the residents to see her
complete it and enjoying the whole atmosphere, I wanted to do it
myself. A few years later I got my chance to run for P.A.L.M.S.
My aim was to raise one thousand pounds which I'm proud to
say I exceeded by raising £1300, but whenever I mentioned to
people that I was running the Marathon they assumed it was for*

Cancer Research. I would explain that I grew up around a lot of the residents that are still there today and would explain the work the charity did for the residents. I even mentioned Jan in a letter to Stephen Fry, himself a sufferer from mental illness. I mentioned the success of her story, as I did to most people who were sponsoring me, and Stephen Fry was kind enough to sponsor me generously. I think that being able to tell the story of Jan helped people to realise the good work the homes could do. Running the marathon was an amazing experience and to be able to run for the residents was a real pleasure.

Whilst I was at school I never got bullied for the work my mum did, but whenever I did mention what my mum did there were always the typical 'spastic' remarks. It never really bothered me, but I remember walking round town with a couple of friends and then little Gwen came and started chatting away with me. Lovely woman, but very hard to get away from when she starts chatting! I chatted with Gwen for a little while whilst she spoke to me about the volunteer work she was doing, then about the college work she was doing; it was always nice to talk to Gwen. When I managed to pry myself away to catch up with my friends and the first thing they said was 'Is that your new girlfriend?' - Just joking of course. I explained she was one of the residents and that she was just telling me what she had got up to recently. My friends' first response was 'Oh.' I think in their mind they expected someone with Down's Syndrome or something of that nature. I think they were quite surprised in their own mind about the appearance of 'mentally ill' people. I would quite often walk past a resident in town and say to whoever I was with that they were a resident, and never did one of my friends expect that the person they just passed was anything but 'normal'. They would always expect to see someone with mental illness coming a mile off, and for me it was all just normal because I'd grown up with it all. Not that I'd change it at all.

It was not only the residents I became attached to, it was also the staff who worked there. With living at Portland Street in the little flat with my mum I often saw the staff, and even now that I'm older I still have some good banter with the staff who are still there. It always made me laugh that I was a well known person to a lot of the residents and even staff for that matter, because I suppose I was always known as 'The Boss's son' and as most people would have some work to do with my mum, I suppose they would always hear about me, so most people knew who I was before I'd met them.

When I was fifteen I asked Dave and Helen if I could do my work experience with them. They agreed, and I think lucky for me that my mum happened to be away for those two weeks. Helen thought I could be best used at The Mill and it was a very enjoyable experience. I'd help with general things such as cleaning, or would play games with the residents; I even helped one or two move rooms. It was a very funny place to work and I can understand why my mum and other staff would stay for so long, because it really was a nice place to be around. I still bump into a few of the residents around town and it is always good to see them and hear how they are getting on. A few years later I had just got back from my summer job and I needed some extra money, so mum said they would pay me to take one of the residents out to play squash or football or whatever we could do. I couldn't believe what I'd just been offered!! To get paid to play squash and get the court paid for. I was more than happy to take that on! I was playing a guy called GB. Now GB has to be one of the fittest blokes I've ever met. He always biked the 16 mile round trip to play squash and to my knowledge whilst he was at college he got a puncture in his bike and couldn't be bothered to change it so he decided to run every day he was at college for the 6 week course. When we were playing squash we both started to become quite good and always wanted to go for longer but would usually play the best of three. The thing that would make me chuckle was that GB never wore shoes. I would ask him if he had trainers to wear, he just said that he preferred to play in bare feet.

I wish I could remember more about my time as a child growing up around the homes, but out of all the experiences with the residents, staff and the around the homes I wouldn't change a thing and truly believe that it has helped turn me into the man I am today.

Anna – a great discovery:

I will never forget the trepidation I felt driving to the Mill House for the first time to start doing some voluntary work. In fact several times during the short drive from Kings Lynn to Gayton I nearly turned back. This was not due to the residents or staff at Mill House or indeed being scared of hard work, in fact I relished in both these aspects; no, it was entirely my own self doubt - would I prove to be a suitable person for what lay ahead?

Not to bore everyone with details, suffice to say I had been somewhat of a 'wild child' and even into adulthood seemed to have a knack of 'messing up'. My dear mother asked Helen if she would mind me coming to the Mill to cook, clean, anything really, as part of the work experience for a counselling course I was doing at the time. I had planned to break it gently to Helen that I was not the best cook but initially I wanted her to think there was nothing in it between me and Jamie Oliver! And I appeased myself with the fact I could clean, which I must say did not fill me full of confidence as it was not too much to offer your future boss.

So here I was driving to Gayton to start my voluntary work, thinking my only credential was that Helen had taken me on as a huge favour to my Mum. I imagined the staff would stick me out of sight and hope I would soon tire of my duties and disappear into the sunset.

This was not the case. Helen embraced me and utilized me wisely. To begin with I cleaned like Cinderella and while doing so became aware that Helen often encouraged various residents to help me, which in hindsight I think was probably her way of assessing how I interacted with them and generally fitted into the Mill House team. I must have passed the 'Helen test' as it was not long before I was no longer a voluntary worker but a real member of the staff team. I also soon realised that with Helen's favour or not, no one would darken the Mill door for long if they did not fit into the ethos of the house. This ethos being that everyone, residents and staff alike, were capable of positive achievements and we were all dedicated to supporting each other in striving towards our goals.

Helen always saw the good qualities in people however deep they were buried, which gave everyone, including me, a chance to blossom. Her attitude encouraged me to go from strength to strength and I did indeed begin to blossom. However, there was one shift I worked that still makes my blood run cold whenever I think about it.
I had not long been a 'real' member of the staff team and it was a glorious sunny day. True to form, Helen was not going to let an opportunity pass for us to go out and soak up the rays, so before I knew it I was in the driving seat of the minibus, which was full to capacity with fifteen of us heading towards Hunstanton for a fun day out.

En route a resident needed to go to the loo so we stopped at a garden centre in Dersingham. The car park was heaving and once in I did feel slightly worried that getting out would be a challenge, but Helen's "anything's possible" attitude was contagious, so in I went. Later, as we left the car park I heard the crunch of metal and realised I had reversed into a car. It was quite a new car and the owner was rather miffed. In fact she was shouting at me, a large vein pulsating in her forehead. I desperately tried to reassure the irate woman that everything would be fine and expressed how sorry I was. Not that I was entirely convinced that everything would be fine, for out of the corner of my eye I could see the younger male residents becoming agitated and instinctively knew they were feeling protective towards me on account of the poor woman's behaviour and that this situation could escalate to a higher level. I had visions of the dented car being only the beginning of a very bad day for the car driver if she did not calm down. So I morphed into my mother and somehow managed to quell the situation. Then I rang the Mill to explain my predicament, convinced I would be handed my P45 immediately when I returned to

Gayton. Not so! Helen gave relevant details to the woman who at this point was hyperventilating, so thankfully quiet, then Helen said to me "Oh well, it's done now, so just carry on and enjoy your day at the beach" Which we all did!

On arriving back at Gayton I was asked to walk to the local garage and collect the Mill House car. One of the residents accompanied me for the exercise. The mechanic at the garage told me to just take the car as the keys were already in it, so I did. I must explain at this point that I had not ever driven this car nor really taken much notice of it, so I was slightly surprised to note there was a baby seat in the back, but with Helen anything's possible and I did not dwell on the matter. The young man who came with me did mumble something which I could not hear properly and he refused to repeat himself; he only ever gave you one opportunity to hear what he said, so we just went ahead and got into the vehicle. The young man tried on a pair of rather smart sunglasses in the glove compartment which really suited him and off we drove to the Mill.

We were greeted by a bemused member of staff whose words were indelibly etched in my brain; "Anna, that's the wrong car!" Initially I thought she was winding me up as I had had an eventful day regarding vehicles, so I flippantly replied "Yes, I just picked a car, any car!" and inadvertently that was exactly what I had done; the only right thing was the colour of the car. Once I had spoken the words I waited for the laughter to follow... it did not! Realisation dawned so I had to retrieve the sunglasses and wheel spin back to the garage. Thankfully only the mechanic was aware of my error and he made sure the next car I took was the correct one, and funnily enough this one did not have a baby seat! So in a seven hour shift I had achieved reckless driving and car theft, good even by my old standards. Anyway, that episode rounded off one of my more memorable work shifts.

My time at the Mill with Dave and Helen at the helm has been the most inspirational and fulfilling period of my life. Helen taught me generosity and enthusiasm and has inspired me and many others to achieve great things and enrich our lives beyond our wildest expectations. It was a very sad day indeed when they left, and they will always be held in the highest esteem and affection by all of us who experienced their unique leadership and guidance.

We had a lot of students pass through our door to do a placement with us as part of their course. We met some wonderful people and most of the time the students helped out a great deal.

John's Story;

I first became aware of the Mill about thirty years ago when Helen and Dave took me on for three months as a Social Work student. An agreement was drawn up between the college, the Mill, my practice teacher and me to achieve various 'learning outcomes'. This required me to examine, assess and evaluate the social work systems employed by Helen and Dave. I needed to consider plans, and what social work methodology they employed.

For my three months' placement I renovated a trailer in the front parking area. Now it might seem I was being exploited but I see it as a happy time during which I learnt a tremendous amount about people. I learnt about seeing people with mental health issues as just that; not people different from 'us'. I went on to work in youth offending for the next twenty-five years. My time at the Mill reinforced my belief that quality comes from caring. It cannot be legislated for or artificially manufactured. Over the past fifteen years or so a culture came from America of quality control which originated in motor car factories to reduce faulty vehicles leaving the factory. Fine. This certainly improved efficiency and workers were controlled by check lists, time and motion etc. That is not quality. Quality cannot be directly measured. The nearest we can get to identifying quality is by noticing when it is absent.

Quality control arrived and fast became part of our work life culture. All well and good in production line systems to improve output, but not in the caring professions. We found ourselves in a culture of value for money. 'Quality' became the Holy Grail. Unfortunately what it achieved was people who worked with people doing less of what was most effective; personal interaction. The emphasis grew toward gathering evidence of our work being cost effective. The growth of computers in our working lives provided Management with the perfect tool to gather this evidence. Money became the controlling factor at the expense of the very thing it was designed to achieve; quality. Workers were pressured to comply with National Standards to ensure 'quality'. What it achieved was qualified, very experienced staff having to see a young person twice a week for six months regardless of whether that intervention was needed other than to tick a box at the expense of not spending time needed with another individual who, because they were not deemed high risk by the tick box system, did not qualify. What was driven out of our work was being able to provide quality intervention. Caring about what we do is the only requirement for quality to exist.

The work at the Mill had genuine quality. It came from people caring. Everything else automatically fell into place. Efficient? Not really if you measured 'time in – product out' thinking. Quality in terms of people growing and being able to exist as happily as their mental health problems would allow? People were encouraged to grow. It was achieved by demonstrating the right way to be. It worked. It reinforced what I already believed and I took that way of working into my professional life. It worked. Eventually the drive towards value for money and the resultant tick box culture ensured we failed. I retired early to get away from what had become a machine chasing the unachievable goal of quality through legislation which completely stifles creativity.

We made up the blurb needed for the college tick boxes. I didn't feel the slightest guilt!

Another student describes her placement at the Mill:-

A good place to start:

My connection to Mill House, Dave and Helen and the residents was through various experiences. I attended fund-raising fetes in the garden, in the summer, with both my girls, carol singing sessions at Christmas and big music festivals. I ran creative writing groups and worked there during a professional degree-level training fieldwork placement. Always, I was very aware that Mill House was a special place where human diversity and individual character were celebrated. The supposed 'divide' between those who were experiencing significant mental health problems and those who were not was never less apparent anywhere I have ever been, before or since. The positive, person-centered ethos was always paramount and there is no doubt that it rubbed off on me.

I'm an OT now, an occupational therapist, or that's what it says on my paperwork. I'm currently working with children with mental health problems and their families. What is an occupational therapist? Well, it seems all OT's find this difficult to define, but from what I can make out, it's a person who, for their job, helps people with a whole range of issues (physical, mental or social) to overcome the challenges in order to lead the most fulfilling life they can, if indeed that is what they want to do. The 'occupational' bit means that the therapeutic tools we therapists use are anything that can ordinarily (or even extraordinarily) occupy a person. This is because our knowledge of that individual (gained by assessment and getting to know them) has provided us with knowledge of exactly which activity (or selection of activities) will help them achieve or overcome. It also means that we help them to maintain or return to the human occupations they would like to continue, having been prevented from carrying out that activity by illness (physical or mental) or disability. It sounds complicated, but it's just supporting and guiding that person to do stuff that helps, with some help to identify what that stuff might be. I'll give you an example of an occupational approach to therapy, from my own experience. When I'm stressed or down in the dumps, I cook something tasty for me and my family. A simple occupation, but when you examine it (OT's describe this as 'activity analysis'), I get so much from it;

Recipe ingredients for 'cooking as a therapeutic activity'

A sense of achievement which improves my self esteem and confidence.

An expression of creativity that gives me a sense of identity both in terms of having creative ability but also in terms of my roles as mother, wife and provider.

A family meal which improves and cements relationships.

Development of concentration, planning, sequencing and fine motor skills.

A purposeful, focused activity that provides a break or distraction from stress or low mood.

An end product in the form of a made from scratch, wholesome, hearty meal, fulfilling one of our basic needs.

I did all this 'occupation for emotional wellbeing' stuff before I learnt about being an OT. I did know that if an activity was fulfilling for me I could use it purposefully. It's just the way I viewed things. I had no idea at that time about making a career out of it. From what I saw though, it was going on at the Mill all the time!

I'll tell you another example of therapeutic occupation, which led to me contributing to the work that happened at Mill House, but also to my subsequent career. When I had any particularly distressing problems, I discovered if I wrote about them, in poetry, I could deal with them better, sometimes even work my way to a solution. The poems were not anything compared to the writings of the great poets of literature, but they were as valuable to me as if they were and I shared many of them with my friends. I talked of how writing out my problems had changed my perspective, or given me hope. One of my wise friends was then *working at Mill House. She was ever one for a great idea and giving people a nudge in the right direction, and she suggested I offer my ideas about writing in the form of workshops at Mill House. She felt sure that Helen and Dave would welcome some volunteer input. As an unemployed single mother of two little girls at the time I was keen to do something that might help me find a career path, so I sat down and wrote a plan for just how these workshops might run. I thought about what I knew of Helen and Dave and their work at the Mill and I tried to plan something that would fit with their whole ethos. I planned to be flexible and adaptable. I presented my ideas to Helen and Dave. They were, of course, typically encouraging and accepting and we worked out the details. I was to offer weekly creative writing groups.*

Each week I turned up at Mill House and explored the medium of writing as a therapeutic tool. I used the works of existing authors and poets to inspire and generate interest. I encouraged the members of the group to write their own pieces and at times got them to work as a team to put a piece of writing together. We were an eclectic group. One member had an English Literature degree and had already written many technically complex and artistic pieces of writing. Another had never learned to read or write, but could skillfully regale you with hilarious or sad stories, full of colourful characters and detailed scenes, all of which I recorded onto audio tape, writing up the transcripts for her later. Another member was only three years old and toddled around the group clutching her little lunch box, keeping herself busy, until Mummy was finished running the group and was ready to take her to pick up her sister from pre-school!

There were aims and goals for the group. It was about boosting confidence, encouraging expression of self, feeding and nurturing creativity, reminiscence and fantasy, making sense of experience, achieving something. It was about connecting with people, finding out about them, learning to work together with them and learning from them. We produced a booklet of Mill House resident writings. Being flexible and adaptable made it work. My group were keen and responsive. I was made to feel very welcome by them and they were very accepting of the presence of my little daughter. In fact her presence provided a connecting point. She was rather cute!

I was inspired. I felt there was something more I could do with this. I took some careers advice, and discovered that what I had been doing was very close to what occupational therapy was and that it could mean a career in mental health. I took a year's access course and continued to conduct the Mill House writing workshops. I went to the University of East Anglia to do an Occupational Therapy degree. In my final year I had to do an elective placement. With some careful planning I was back at the Mill, for eight weeks. I implemented a temporary occupational therapy service which included assessment and intervention and therapeutic activities which aimed at promoting independent living skills, emotional well-being, confidence and self esteem. I set up a 'soup club', arts and crafts activities and revisited the writing group. I also carried out general community support home support worker duties.

The writing group evolved into a trip out to somewhere in the mini bus to get inspired before coming back to write up our experiences. Once again with that opportunist 'can do' attitude, other residents who did not take part in the writing joined us for the visits. I'd never driven a mini-bus before, but it was the group participants who helped me to feel confident about this and I have fond memories of driving down country lanes, chatting and sharing jokes with the group members.

Soup club was an exercise in independent living skills and another wonderful social opportunity. I pitched it to the residents and asked for a volunteer one lunch time a week. They would have to choose a soup recipe, plan and shop for it, cook it and serve it to the other residents with whatever level of support they needed from me. There's nothing like a big vat of soup to bring people together. The residents were so kind and appreciative to those who took turns. And the chefs for the day all committed their time and energy without reservation. It generated quite a buzz and some great healthy lunch soups. We were not short of volunteers over the eight weeks.

Although my mini OT service had to conform to the university requirements and of course, to the needs and wishes of the residents, as well as to the remit of Community Support Homes, as a placement opportunity for me it was luxurious. Once again this is because of the congruence between OT philosophy, Mill House ethos and my own beliefs and principles. It was a harmonious blend which produced good results.

Dave and Helen were incredibly appreciative and kind about my input, as was my friend who had recommended me and then supervised me during my fieldwork placement. I am the one who has to thank them and all of the residents I came into contact with. My experience with Mill House was life-affirming. It set me on both my career and personal development course and provided me with an excellent arena to cultivate my skills, understanding and knowledge. I learned so much from those I cooked with, wrote with, shopped with, painted with, travelled with, drank coffee with, laughed and cried with. I see many of them about town and it is a pleasure to catch up with them and remember those days. I have not mentioned any of you by name, but I hope that each of you can remember those times and are aware that I have been privileged to know you.

Helen's opinions once more:

Many people can achieve qualifications and pass exams. Although I would never undermine these skills, they are no more important, in my opinion, than a person with life skills, common sense, compassion and an ability to listen if the role is to support people in residential care and in the community. My message to anyone wanting to work in Community Support Homes would be; "Don't work here if you're lazy or have poor motivation".

It's a great place to work with energy and fun on offer. We needed a variety of staff so that residents could find personalities that they felt comfortable with. We needed people from a variety of backgrounds with a variety of life skills to draw on.

When we employed Netty, she had been working on a barn conversion opposite the Mill House. Every day she climbed ladders and laboured as one of the men. To me, it suggested that she could work as part of a team, get her hands dirty and have the courage to work in an environment that most women would pass by. Her interview was held by me and a couple of residents. Netty was impressed that we had a handsome black doctor on our interview panel. He was in fact a resident. It interested me greatly how people often make assumptions. We gave her the job even though her knowledge of mental health was very limited and she had no experience in this field of work. I always felt that people could learn if they were interested enough. It was good giving people a new career direction or a new personal challenge.

Staff needed respect for themselves and others regardless of creed, colour or problems. They needed a level head and endless energy. Provided that a new worker could prove this, they were often employed. New workers needed to show that they really wanted to do this type of work, as jobs would be offered to people with no qualifications or experience. Some people coming for interviews with previous experience would have fixed ideas or a contamination of thoughts and ideas that would not fit into our 'free' way of thinking. Residents would gain confidence and build self-esteem needed for any future success, providing the staff had the skills and ability to help them along their journey of recovery. Sometimes this was the ability to listen. So often people can find their own solutions in the right forum. They need time to talk, discover, reflect and think in an environment that allows this to happen.

We tried hard not to create a 'them and us' situation. It would be unrealistic to say that we were equal within our living and working environment. How could we be? We had a job to do and working relationships were important. We were all being paid to do a job to the best of our ability. However, this did not make us any different in terms of having human needs. I used to relay this to residents who felt that others were more important by saying "We all poo on the same pot, we were created in the same way and we are all going to end up in the same place. We all have different skills and abilities and we are no better than the next person".

Boundaries between staff and residents were at times cloudy. I would promote working relationships rather than friendships, although since leaving Mill House I have residents that I now call friends and hope to keep them as friends for a very long time. At times I would say to the staff "Would you pick this person as your friend if you were to meet in a pub or a club? Would you expect an equal give and take relationship or be able to confide in that person?" Mostly they would say not. Some residents are engaging, intelligent and interesting, but that doesn't mean you would necessarily want them as your friend. Our working role is to help residents move on, make their own friends and not create false relationships that have no real future or sustainability as this is unrealistic and unfair. We had to be careful whist working alongside somebody that we didn't lose sight of our aims and outcomes and that our own needs were not getting in the way. I think most people working in care have their own unrecognised needs. It might be the need to feel needed or the need to prove to oneself or others that you are worthwhile. I think if people look deep within themselves and are honest they would probably discover why they work in the caring field.

Besides it being a great place to be, separation of my own life, family and working all became a bit tied up together. It was for many years difficult to separate. It was a lifestyle choice for Dave and I. Our boys had no choice other than to fit into the life on offer and the life we had chosen. We didn't even discuss with the boys what line of work we were in (in the early days I don't think we knew ourselves!). Saving lost souls and the 'worried well' and the 'needy' springs to mind. I was surprised one afternoon when my eldest, Shane, came home from school and he had to write an essay about what his parents did. Looking rather confused he asked "Do we run a bed and breakfast?" I explained that we looked after people with problems and gave him a few simple examples. Although, perhaps, the boys should have known that the people sharing their home had problems, we clearly hadn't ever made the problems a primary importance. It was always people first, problems second. Shane was eleven when he asked that question. As he and Lee got older they became more aware of some residents' difficulties but took everyday events in their stride. They had a wonderful childhood living within the main house that housed most of the residents.

Periodically Dave and I would feel the need to indulge ourselves in some ordinary family life. We decided Monday teatimes would be our night to sit around our own table and eat a family meal together; quality time. I would prepare a family favourite. The boys would eat their dinner and then say "Can we go back into the main house now?" They would trot back through, leaving Dave and I looking bemused, so we would just follow them through. The buzz of the main house was always a draw for us all.

A Scrabble game at the kitchen table was always 'very competitive', especially if Donna was playing. People would crash out on the big sofas in front of the wood burner, watching the box; usually with the St. Bernard or spaniel at their feet. Someone would always be munching something weird and wonderful from the kitchen. One of our ladies enjoyed jam and marmite sandwiches or the odd biscuit dunked in a cup of soup. There's no accounting for individual taste; everyone just did their own thing.

Staff Meetings:

Every week the Mill staff would get together for a staff meeting. Dave would take the meeting minutes and I would chair. We had an agenda book which was kept in the office for staff to put a quick heading of an issue they would like to bring up at the next meeting. As in the residents' meeting some would talk too much and some staff would say very little. I was, at times, a complete pest. Ady and Gemma used to have private bets on how long I would discuss a subject, although I didn't know this at the time! There were some very serious issues to discuss and work out as a team, especially when dealing with people with personality disorders who needed boundaries that were clear and firm. Alongside the practical and serious discussions were the laughs. Everyone in the staff gang had a wonderful sense of humour, and at many meetings we would literally cry tears of laughter. The energy was high from our 'off the wall' staff team, and we would inevitably catch up with each other's private lives and the calamities they went through – and there were always a few! This was a good forum for letting off steam, sharing thoughts and ideas, bonding together and establishing camaraderie which I think we achieved. We were a very tight group.

I'm sure it was a great tonic to us all, considering our work was not easy; never a minute to spare and never knowing what we would be faced with. We were not robots and had our own difficulties to deal with.

To help staff with their working practice and self preservation individual time was always on offer with myself, Dave or a senior member of staff. It was a time to offer a confidential service to help unload personal, private and work related concerns. I would tell staff that it was like having time with a vomit pot; anything and everything could pour out. It was also a creative exploring time to help maximise the care plans for residents. Each staff member had responsibility for at least a few residents as we worked on a key worker system. We would look at their files and explore ideas that might help engage the residents in question with more things to do. It might be looking at personal hygiene problems, relations with others; the list would be endless. At times the staff needed more than I could offer. We paid for outside supervision with a counsellor or therapist of their choice. Working within a job that has so many personal demands, it's important to be 'untangled' yourself. We need to be kept mentally and physically well to do the job well. I always saw the staff as the anchors; if they were not safe and sound the whole ship would start to rock.
I wish other industries and caring professions would look after

their staff. It's such false economy not to.

The loyalty and commitment from the staff never ceased to impress me, we were so lucky having such great people to spend our working life with. They gave the job their 'all'.

Every resident was assigned a key worker. The residents did not choose who they had as a key worker. This was not because we wanted to be bossy; we wanted to give staff a realistic number of people, especially as other workload commitments had to be taken into consideration (i.e. if staff were already in charge of medication or health and safety).

Sometimes we felt that a complex teenager would work well with a specific staff role model. It might be that a resident who had been out of control with their illness needed a very experienced mental health worker who could keep a close eye on their mental health state. The role was not about building a special relationship with one staff member, nor was it to become a dependent relationship in any way. The role of a key worker was to put a care plan together with the resident, amending it when necessary. The information system was put in place for every resident. A snapshot of their life was collected by the key worker and put on file. These files were shared at staff meetings to help formulate a week's plan suitable for the individual. All staff were responsible for getting to know all of the individuals living in the house, therefore creating no dependent relationships on one staff member and allowing a resident to develop relationships with all staff members. So, in a nutshell, information was gathered by the key worker and shared amongst the staff to give the team a good understanding of all residents and their needs.

The importance of staff and resident relationships goes without saying. One resident, Karen gives her views on just how important they are:-

I believe that the measure of any community lies in the quality of the relationships between the inhabitants, and in Community Support Homes this was of particular importance. Developing appropriate boundaries and healthy relationships was a steep learning curve which, although it took place over years, was constantly aimed towards achieving.

Many (but my no means all) of the residents had experienced damaging and destructive models of relating to others and needed to be exposed to healthier examples of communication and behaviour in relationships. This started at the top, if you like, with the committed affection between Helen and Dave being expressed in terms of mutual respect. As with any relationship they had their share of tiffs and disagreements and it certainly wasn't a stuffy or repressed relationship, but there was no doubt in anyone's mind that they were made for each other. This respect set the tone for relationships between staff and residents. We knew we mattered, we knew we had significance in the house but we also knew that it was expected that we should show the same courtesy to others. For some people being treated this way perhaps for the first time in their lives was a healing experience, especially for those alienated by society. Others bucked against it and would test the limits to the extreme.

Many, I am told, criticised the work that went on at the Mill for having no boundaries, but in fact nothing could have been further from the truth. True, the setting of parameters was a skill that was honed over a period of time, and in the early stages this had certainly not been perfected, but the goal to provide safe limits was successful in the longer term with both staff and residents secure in where they stood.

Communication was in fact so clear, direct and straightforward that a list of rules pinned up on a board somewhere would have been totally redundant. This openness and honesty gave each person a sense of security. There were no hidden agendas or insecurity although this truthful communication was expressed for the most part in a way that could be received positively. To put it another way, if your behaviour was unacceptable the opportunity to turn it around would be given in all but the most serious of misdemeanours. Very little time was spent on negatives, and bucket loads of praise, encouragement and affirmation were given for positive steps taken, no matter how small.

Helen and Dave played a large part in the lives of the residents and both in their ways had about them a huge presence. Helen's energy, enthusiasm and sense of humour could lift the atmosphere of the house the minute she walked through the door. True, some would run for cover, but on the whole she was like a human magnet. Dave had his own powerful influence and could communicate with just a look. His contribution was enormous, and his point of view put across with just a few words was invaluable. As a role model for the male residents he was second to none and he remains one of the most respected individuals I know.

Both Helen and Dave could have easily found themselves with a problem of dependency in their relationships with their residents. Over the years, however, they developed the ability to empower those in their care to build healthy relationships with family and friends and to keep a balance of support and independence which helped minimise this potential pitfall.

As someone who has lived in Community Support Homes under Helen and Dave's care with varying degrees of support I have found that I have been treated not as a client, service user or even particularly as a resident but above all as a human being with the same needs and right to respect and dignity as anyone else. My experience has enriched and transformed my values and attitudes to others. I shall always be grateful to Helen, Dave and the very special team they led and inspired.

I'd like to thank Karen and others for such positive feedback about myself, Dave and all of our staff team. However, we certainly didn't get it right all the time, especially in the early years. We did try to do the best for everyone and, I think people understood this, but hindsight is a great thing.

Although we always strived toward clear communication we would often meet others who didn't have the skill and we would be left to trial and error. The problems usually arose because of illness or background and we would have to be creative in our search to find ways to communicate. An example follows;

He was 17 years old and tucked silently up in the corner of the local psychiatric ward. His skin was pale, his hair jet black, he was very thin and showed no emotion. I was introduced to Mick by his social worker. He had been admitted into the unit with thought disorders and a drug induced psychosis. Family and friends could no longer cope with his outrageous outbursts and at times volatile behaviour. However, he looked a broken person with virtually no communication skills. I did what I usually did in these situations. I talked, laughed, told him about the Mill and told him it was like living in 'Fawlty Towers'. I invited him to come for a coffee with us. I told him I would pick him up the next week on the Monday. I told him to ring me if this was not OK.

My technique of talking to people, engaging with them if they gave me any positive eye contact or verbal communication, became quite a skill. I felt confident enough to read their body language and many other non verbal communications, to engage with them at some level as to where they were at. I wanted to leave everybody with a positive feeling, hope, encouragement and an underlying message that they would be 'OK'. Being ever the optimist I really believed this, regardless of anyone's presentation. For the record, Mick did come for a coffee that Monday, and eventually moved in to the Mill where he became a confident, self assured young man and went on to gain professional employment.

CHAPTER SIXTEEN

Extracts From the Daily Records;

A.m. - ****** walking round in only his underpants. Suggested he put some clothes on. Was told to f*** off and he is insisting he hates all staff and all the residents and is not going to take his medication.
P.m. – Same resident – fully clothed now and has taken his medication. Fully engaged in a game of Monopoly with three other residents. Appears happy and relaxed.
Staff intervention for this situation – a word in his ear about what he has to offer our community and the effects his negative behaviour has on himself and others. All is well until the next time! Negativity is here to be challenged.

****** continues masturbating while holding a conversation. Told to come and have a chat once he has relieved himself as conversation now is inappropriate.

Residents getting cross with ****** She has yet again lost her voice. This has become a charade as there doesn't appear to be anything wrong with her voice. Staff to engage her in positive activity without discussing her voice.

The summer weather seems to be making some of the men in the house frisky. ******* complained that ******** was 'wanking' in the sitting room. I asked ******** if it was true and he said he was only pretending. I suggested that if he felt the need to relieve himself the privacy of his own bedroom would be best.

******'s dad died today. Lots of support and TLC needed.

******* has dressed in bow tie and crisp white shirt and jacket and has gone to town. He is convinced that he is a millionaire and solicitors are withholding his money. He returned later having had a very successful day being a passenger in various BMWs on test drives while waiting for his millions to arrive. He is planning what cars to purchase and is convinced it will happen and it's not a delusion.

*******achieved her first bus trip today unaccompanied. Staff met her at the bus station. We have all congratulated her.

*******'s gone out with her boyfriend. *******'s gone to her cousin's for the night and says she may stay an extra day if it rains. Everybody really enjoyed dressing up for the Indian evening. We feasted on lovely food that so many people helped to prepare. We sang and danced using kitchen equipment for improvised instruments.

******* needed a lot of encouragement to get out and cut the grass while several others were weeding and planting.

******* is still insisting he can smell BO but can't identify who it is and would like us to 'do something about it' I have explained that he is the only resident who can smell it but he still insists we do something.

A group has really enjoyed apple picking in Sandringham.

******* climbed onto the flat roof with his butterfly net as he could see a bird perched in the yew tree. The bird flew past him a few times and he took several swipes at it but sadly to no avail. I persuaded him to come down, however, as it all looked very hazardous and being such a big chap I was frightened he might fall through the roof.

******* is having a day chilling out, listening to music and swinging in the hammock.

Hippy day in the garden has been a great success. Sal entertained us by playing the guitar and singing. Annie painted several peoples' faces in the teepee we made. Nick made home made lemonade and we ate BBQ food. The sun shone and everyone spent the day in the garden.

Five of us went to buy French bread for lunch. On our return to the car a blue budgie was sat on the roof. I opened the car and took the bird inside. We have brought him back to the Mill. Lee is delighted. He has called the bird Norman. Norman is now sitting very happily in an old Fisher Price aeroplane in Lee's bedroom. None of us like cages so he will live with Lee in his bedroom.

******* told me today that she had been to the chemist to buy a suppository as she has been suffering from constipation. She said it was very difficult to swallow and it made her 'gag'. I said I thought she may have put it in the wrong end but not to worry. If the problem continues we will organise a Doctor's appointment if she wants one.

******* had problems watching Holly today (the Mills St Bernard). She insisted on chewing a dead rabbit that was squashed into the tarmac on the road and refused to budge until she had had her fill.

An irate man from the village came to the Mill today and said Holly had done a big poo in his gateway and the walker had not cleaned it up. I said I was very sorry and would follow him home in my car to pick the poo up. When we arrived at his house there was no poo. He was confused as to where the poo had gone. I returned to the Mill and walking in the gate was Jo and Holly. I asked if the dog had poo'ed in somebody's gateway and she said yes but didn't have a bag with her so had asked the butcher for a bag and then went back and cleaned it.

I was really proud of the gang today. Gwen and crew went round the village and down by the stream and collected bags of litter that people had dropped. They have piled bin bags full of their collections ready for the local farmer who has agreed to dispose of them. What a great contribution to the village!

As you can see by some of the records kept there was never a dull moment. As the years progressed daily records had to be kept as a government requirement. In fact pieces of paper had to be kept about everything and at times I felt we were being buried alive with paper exercises – it drove us mad. When we started Mill House we didn't have staff, we just lived as a big family. We didn't have an office – we didn't need one. By the time we left I can't imagine how many trees we used to satisfy various organisations that we were doing our job properly. We had a business manager, office staff, floor manager and 35 staff members, and although I enjoyed the day to day challenges, still I felt claustrophobic and restrained by so many new requirements and changing systems. It was at times hard to get on with doing what I felt our job was, and that was working with people, not ticking boxes, playing lip service and feeling crushed by the system. As for health and safety, that had become beyond a joke. I know at times throughout my 25 years at Mill House I have not always recognised danger, but we had to put up signs to tell people they may hit their head, fall down a step, that the hot water tap was hot and signs for every possible thing that might happen. Risk assessments now had to be done before anyone went anywhere on a trip. Recently a risk assessment had to be done on a cat! The world has gone crazy. The people who live at community support homes are bright, intelligent people; they are not children or very elderly, and while they live in the homes as their place of residence they know that the hot tap is hot! It's their home. One of the most ridiculous things we had to do was to put a ramp outside Adrian Lodge. The angle of the concrete ramp had to slope gently up to the door for wheelchair users – I'm all for equal opportunities but anyone visiting the house using a wheelchair would have to stay in the hallway as the doorways were too small for wheelchairs, as were the toilet and bathrooms. We couldn't accept people with physical disabilities because none of the properties were deemed to be 'fit for purpose', and they weren't. The only use the ramp had was to give our handyman the job of replacing the handrail several times after the staff driving the minibus knocked it off as the ramp and rail were so close to the gateway. We did have some terrible staff drivers! The residents who were allowed to drive the vehicles were far more competent!

Looking after yourself and your staff team has always felt very important to me. I do have to confess that looking after others first has not always been helpful to meeting my own needs, and I have at times neglected myself and paid the price.

As time progressed in my working life I became more and more aware that I should not shoulder responsibility that was not mine. I would try my best to rescue everyone from their emotional grief and pain. I realized quite early on that if I was going to survive in this job I would have to learn not to take on board everyones' problems. I needed to create relationships that would work for both sides. When feeling a little worn out one time my dear social worker friend Maggie said "Helen, you must try and be a little more selfless and more selfish to survive this workload" I was grateful for this advice; words of wisdom that I have passed on to other workers, carers and parents.

In my experience the balance between doing too much or not enough is a tough decision to make. Sometimes we get it wrong. Some residents would go to extremes to prove a point, have their say or defend themselves. On one occasion I had given firm words to a woman who was intent on her own self destruction. The morning after I had had these words about her destructive behaviour I went to her room to find out where she was as she hadn't come downstairs. After calling and knocking on her door I told her I was going in. Two eyes looked at me from beneath the duvet. I had a one way conversation and turned to leave, stressing that I was sorry she didn't want to talk to me. As I turned to leave, the duvet came down. She had stitched her mouth up with black thread. The neatness immediately struck me; there were herringbone stitches across her mouth. Tiny knots were tied at each end of her lips. "What on earth have you done that for?" I said "I will have to go and get a pen and paper so you can write down why you've done such a thing to yourself". I went to the office, got a pen and some paper and told Dave what she had done, and sensibly he followed with a pair of nail scissors. How silly was I to think that it was the time and place to write down why she had done it! I think I was in shock and was flabbergasted. Luckily, Dave had the sense (and courage) to free her sewn lips. She could have choked while I stood confused as to why she had done such a thing. I rang her consultant later that morning and told him what had happened. He asked me what I thought needed to happen now. I said nothing; I felt that we needed to talk through the woman's actions and move on. Her past history had suggested that she always 'upped the anti' when things upset her and usually this would lead to another hospital admission. I really wanted her to break this destructive pattern of behaviour. She did, eventually. She moved on into her own home, became very competent at needlecraft, homemaking and cooking. Sometimes we just had to take risks and ride a storm!

CHAPTER SEVENTEEN

Sometimes I felt that the system let us and the residents down. This feeling evolved quite strongly in our latter years. An example would be the following:-

An ex-resident phoned me one day from America. She had been living there with her partner for the past couple of years. He had recently left her and she was going through a really tough time, having had a recent miscarriage. Her world was falling apart. Her partner was in the American forces and she had felt set up for life, but had found herself under section in an American psychiatric hospital. Her key worker had spoken to me on the phone and said that the young lady would be coming back to the UK as soon as she was well enough. I asked them to keep me informed. I also had an informal chat with the local Social Services department about her. I brought up the fact that the young woman was soon due back from America and that supported accommodation may be needed for her and we could work together to achieve this. Our Alternative to Hospital Bed that was paid for and used by Social Services could surely be assigned as an emergency placement, giving her a safe place to be while her mental health was assessed. I thought to be safe they might even take the young woman straight to hospital. The American hospital rang on a couple of occasions, stating that she wanted to come back to Mill House. I explained that although in principal this would not be a problem, it would have to be sorted out with the local Community Mental Health Team as they had control of the ATH Bed. The American charge nurse explained that communication with the Social Services department had been very difficult and they didn't want to engage with the problems she was having. One morning the phone rang; it was a friend of the young woman. She said that a support worker had taken her to Kings Lynn and booked her into a 'shady' Bed and Breakfast. She had visited Adrian Lodge that night but the staff on duty were new and didn't know her and the house was particularly quiet that night. She saw only one familiar face, Ady, but didn't know him that well either. Ady made her a cup of tea and in his normal cheery way said "Alright, Sarah?" She told him yes. When I asked him about how she looked and what she said he described her as looking very distant and being very quiet. This young lady died of a heroin overdose that first night home in the Bed and Breakfast. The stand-in manager of Social Services found it hard to look me in the eye the day I tried to engage him in conversation about her death. I'm sure he was 'protecting confidentiality', which was always a good ploy to keep outsiders from prying into things considered to be none of their business. He did seem shocked when I told him that it had been many years since the young woman had touched heroin, that she had many qualifications, that she had been offered a place at university until recent events had thrown her into a fragile mental state. Heroin, I'm sure, was used as her way out. The pain, loneliness and despair were too much for her. Why didn't anyone let me know of her return? Were her parents told? Was anyone she knew told? Was the Section in America taken off so as to allow her to fly back to whoever she knew, knowing Social Services would pick her up, assess the situation and make the appropriate care for this vulnerable young woman? One would have thought so. The answers to some of my questions I shall never know.

I felt attitudes had changed in the professional field and we were often left abandoned and unsupported as were our residents, or at least that's how it felt. I have an example (but believe me there could have been many more) about a young woman who remains in a secure unit. The incident that I shall tell you about led to a disagreement between the learning disability team and the mental health team, as neither felt her to be their responsibility after the serious incident that had occurred. What it boiled down to, in my mind, was that neither team wanted to have the expense of funding her out of their budgets, and I felt her well being was less important than the funding issues.

It was 8am on a Saturday morning when a staff member, Jo, rang to say that the fire brigade was on the way as the Mill House was on fire. Dave was at the Mill within a couple of minutes. The residents gathered together in the car park. It was a freezing cold

Helen Morrell

day and most of them were in their night attire as Saturday was usually a 'chill out' day. Some were more traumatized than others, having been coaxed along the smoke filled corridor. All but one resident was accounted for, until she appeared round the corner of the building. Dave met her eyes and quietly asked if she had set fire to her bedroom. She said "Yes, I lit paper in my bin and then went to the village shop" The fire brigade completed their job and were gone after a couple of hours. The resident was handed over to the police. Dave and I asked for her to be charged with arson. We spent the rest of the day reassuring residents and bringing things back to some normality. Smoke damage was heavy in one of the upstairs areas. The resident's room was gutted, and floorboards had been burnt through, along with curtains, the bed and furniture. One corner cupboard was okay; this held some personal belongings. Social Services were informed about what had happened and we said that the woman could not return under any circumstances. We had to be sure that the other twenty residents were safe. The police rang to say that she had been assessed and it was deemed that there were no mental health issues. She was free to leave and asked us to collect her. We said no and gave the reason why, and that's where the battle began. The Social Services team on duty said they had talked to a senior team leader and that if we didn't take her back we would be in breach of our contract and that we were responsible for the resident. They said that was what we were being paid for and if anything happened to her we would be responsible. What a crazy situation! We continued to battle with any service who would listen. We might as well have saved our breath to cool our porridge.

By now it was late into Saturday night and we had refused to collect her from the police station. They were now giving me a really hard time. I kept explaining the situation. It wasn't a safe place for her to stay, she now had no room, and other residents were terrified as were staff. At midnight the police drove onto the shingle and let the resident out of the car before driving off. What were we going to do? The young woman did not have the capacity to realise fully the consequences of her actions. We were not angry with her. This woman had had a life that would make most people's hair stand on end. She had very little regard for herself and others, she had no ability at building or sustaining relationships, and she was not listened to. She carried unresolved pain, anger and frustration; was it surprising she set light to her bin? She lived in a world where the rules were confusing. I visited an outpatient's appointment with her before the fire. We met with one of her mental health social workers and a consultant. The young woman was asked to wait outside while we had a little chat. The chat was more like a flirtation between the social worker and the consultant. It was pathetic. I enquired what action was going to be taken, as the young woman was claiming to have voices in her head, difficulties sleeping and felt agitated. She had recently taken herself off to London, booked into a B & B, forgot where it was and was found confused by the police who sent her home in a taxi which we paid for. So already there were signs that she was not well or happy.

After a while she knocked on the Consultant's door and asked if he was ready to see her. He replied, that no, it wouldn't be necessary. I was as gob smacked as her. I said to him as he closed the door again "She is upset and wants to talk to you," to which he replied that I was to take her home and he would increase her medication. I left, leaving the Consultant and Social Worker to continue talking about 'important things'. Is it really surprising this young woman set fire to our house?

After days of talking to various professionals and assigning a worker to watch her round the clock she was sent to a secure unit under the care of the learning disability team. They listened to us, they talked and listened to her; at last a really respectful and helpful team came to our aid. We all paid a high emotional price for trying to look after this young woman. The mental health system really let us down. They held the power, and I have no doubt that if they had worked a little harder the outcome could have been healthier for us all. We didn't make an insurance claim for the thousands of pounds worth of damage. We didn't get extra pay for the 24hr staff cover to keep our other residents safe. You people who were involved and able to make decisions made us all pay in many ways.

I do not know why the new system, which has been in place over the last few years, has changed so much. I know there are big financial restraints. But morale throughout the service seems low. Negativity has replaced positive thinking. Blame has become a ready tool. Some system workers seem to resent the fact that we enjoyed our work, our challenges and our achievements, and that we had proactive personalities and wanted our residents to have quality of life. That we built relationships and wanted each and every person leaving in our care to remember the good times we shared together and to continue building their lives.

A lot of the system seems incapable of this as a concept. I am sorry if I offend the workers who put their energy and effort into their clients. I know there are many good people left in the system doing great work with residents such as ours. Thank you for your help and support. I know some of you also feel let down, unsupported and undermined, and I am truly sorry that it is the way it is. It doesn't need to be this way, but contamination of attitude and negative thinking is easily passed from one to another. Are you one of those people? If so, think again. Enjoy the people you work with, look for positive outcomes and lift your own heart and soul in the meantime.

During a local placement one of our ex workers told me that she was advised by a senior professional that one of her first learning outcomes was to forget everything she had learnt from me and Dave. I found these words sad. Did she really have to forget respect and dignity for others, and moral responsibility, kindness and care for everybody, equal opportunities, enjoyment and job satisfaction? These are only a few of the values that our philosophy was based on. It seemed a shame that she was being asked to leave all these things behind. I'm not sure what was going to replace them! She soon left her training because she said it was because of what she learnt at Community Support Homes that she was eager to learn more.

CHAPTER EIGHTEEN

Life is full of 'colour' and events happy and sad; whenever possible I like to smile and move on. I look back at the next scenario and smile to myself. It would have been a sketch suitable for 'Fawlty Towers'.

The phone rings, it's the Mill. Dave is delayed in Norwich and can't get back to meet and greet the relatives of a young woman who has recently moved in. The only staff member at the Mill is Mary, and she has an urgent dental appointment that she can't miss. I tell Mary that I will be down in a few minutes. We are living at a bungalow now, a couple of minutes drive from the Mill. Luckily we have a plumber working in the airing cupboard fixing the new immersion heater. I have a slipped disc in my back following a game of squash and can't walk. For the second time in a week I have to ask for the plumber's help. On his first visit, his head in and out of the bottom of the airing cupboard, he watches me crawl along the hall to the bathroom. He said "Oh dear, is there anything I can do?" "Yes," I said, "please get me a bowl from the kitchen, I'm going to be sick" This was in the early days of the disc slipping and the pain was not funny. The plumber looked uncomfortable and embarrassed. Well, after the call from the Mill I yet again needed his assistance. I was not in as much pain at this point, but my legs didn't seem to want to hold me properly and I couldn't sit down. The only comfortable way round was to crawl. I asked the plumber if he would mind taking me down to the Mill in his van as I needed to be on duty. His face was again a picture; he was a man of few words. We got out to the van and I couldn't get in, well not in a sitting position. I landed up with my bottom stuck in the air facing his windscreen, head down on the seat looking as if I was praying. I can't imagine what his face looked like; I'm only grateful we weren't stopped by the police!

I find this whole event ridiculous looking back on it, but at the time I don't remember thinking anything of it. A job had to be done and so off I went. Residents at the Mill were really great in their support if any staff members were unwell. In fact some were more helpful than they would have been normally. The gang paid little attention to me crawling around, and this was quickly perceived as normal. It might have been normal to the residents, but our visitors looked confused when I greeted them at the front door on my hands and knees announcing that my name was Helen and the owner and manager of the Mill.

As I'm sure I've mentioned, residents came from all walks of life. The wealthy parents of a young woman resident from Hertfordshire came in their own plane to visit her, and to show her aunt where she was living. I, as the proprietor, crawled along the floor with my bad back welcoming them in for a cup of tea. I would have loved a snapshot of their faces but I didn't even think about it at the time. I can't imagine what I must have looked like with my wide bottom waddling in front, expecting them to follow. All went well with the visit and we had lots of laughs. Their daughter made us tea on my instruction which they were suitably impressed with; "She isn't usually very helpful," they commented. They were ready to catch a taxi back to the airfield when one of our male residents who was a 'little high' to say the least popped in. A truly lovely lad if you know him, but he does suffer with mood swings. On this occasion Mum and Auntie were admiring the kitchen beams on their way out. First of all the lad talks loudly to himself. I suggest a few of my distraction techniques to send him on his way to do something else but he is responding to none of my good ideas. Instead he goes up to Mum and Aunt and shouts that he used to 'eat Mars bars out of his mother's fanny'. I'm not sure the well bred, well spoken ladies quite understood his strong Geordie accent thankfully, and they left without further ado.

I guess that mental health doesn't always inflict itself on the people with poor inadequate parenting and deprived backgrounds. I remember thinking on many occasions what on earth went wrong? Why has this happened? How could this mental torture inflict itself on this picture book family, where everything seems so perfect? The cruel reality is that it does. The question remains, is it nature or nurture? That I don't know.

It is cruel and unfair without discrimination, in my experience - the pain that parents, partners, children, husbands and wives have gone through, trying to make sense of what went wrong and why illness struck, when all seemed so well is very apparent.

We had many high achievers; some of our residents came from private schools and professional jobs. We had accountants, teachers, nurses, university lecturers to name a few. Mental illness is known to strike one in every three people at some level and at some time in a person's life, and as we are all individuals the course of events can vary considerably. The repair and healing process has no defined time. What triggers a relapse into another episode of ill health cannot always be measured or predicted. There is no pure science in dealing with mental illness, so when loved ones came to me asking "How long?" I could never say for certain, which may have seemed unsatisfactory. I would try my best to explain our process and procedure, to reassure them that a recovery model was in place and time was needed. When I say a recovery model, it wasn't a standardised instruction sheet. Each person had a care plan drawn up by their key worker, myself or Dave. We would spend time discussing areas of need, ways forward and how to increase the residents' self esteem and confidence. We would look at getting a life balance in place for each resident, which the staff team would encourage and support. All day every day each person in our care was supported with their daily needs. These would vary greatly for each individual and could be forever changing depending on how a person was feeling.

It's hard to explain the complexity of working with each and every individual. I loved my job so much that in 25 years there was never a morning I didn't want to get up. I'm sure some people would envy this. Each day would excite me. A new resident – a new challenge. I travelled to different hospitals around the country to meet potential new residents who needed support once they were discharged from hospital. I visited prisons, adolescent assessment units and secure units. Sometimes my visits tested my own insecurities. I remember on one occasion Dave and I had gone to visit a potential referral who was in a women's prison in Essex. The environment there was old fashioned and had a real feeling of oppression. I seem to have sensitivity around how places feel, and to me this place did not feel good. The social worker involved with this young woman took us down a bleak corridor and into a cell that he was using as a temporary office. The three of us sat in private discussing the young woman's future needs, when alarms started ringing and the doors were automatically locked. As soon as we were confined I felt trapped inside this cell, with the bars automatically closing off all doors along the corridor. We were in a 'lock down' situation. It was a horrible feeling. The social worker said that they didn't last long, but by this time I could hardly breathe. I couldn't quite believe that we were sitting cramped together in this tiny box called a cell. I felt ready to have a panic attack, and God knows how I didn't because my imagination was running riot! I felt so hot, and I'm sure the social worker could see how freaked out I was. Although the experience was ghastly it gives you an insight to how it could feel at first hand having no control even if the building was on fire.

I always found it fascinating to see how people in these jobs cooperated with each other. I enjoyed meeting all the different consultants and staff who worked at these units. Mostly they were very nice people with a high level of respect, knowledge and motivation to ensure a good standard of care and after care for their client or patient. Occasionally I would meet self important 'jobs worth' professionals, but I would try to get them on my side so as to have a productive working relationship which was of the utmost importance when the handover of someone's care was taking place. I liked working as part of a team. I always felt so proud of what we had to offer. It was unique in so many ways. We offered a whole new life experience to people. Their growth and change as individuals was so rewarding to watch, and I always felt a sense of achievement. My energy was my strength. I am an optimistic person who feels very strongly that each individual should be given every chance to recover, rebuild their lives and move on.

Regrets:

If I could turn back the clock it would be when I was helping a reluctant young woman with the dishes one night. She could be described as a stroppy teenager. I still remember the tarnished skin from her waist to her knees; the result of being left for days as a baby without a nappy change – a fairly good indication of her earlier years!

I had ignored for some time the abuse she was hurling at me as we stood at the sink. "Bitch, f***ing cow" and so on. It was to go on some time with me not reacting at all. Suddenly as if from nowhere I lifted the large pan of water from my sink and poured it all over her head. I couldn't believe what I had done and neither could she. Sadly my lack of control had managed to spoil the trifle that a resident had made earlier. I was not proud of my behaviour. I said sorry and we were soon back on speaking terms. I don't know what came over me.

I was driving home one day from one of our outings to Fakenham Market. We always had a bag of chips each to munch on the way home. On this occasion I had eaten a couple of soused herrings from the wet fish shop, therefore declined my portion of chips. The smell of the chips covered with salt and vinegar was divine.

One young woman sitting behind me kept feeding me with her chips as we drove home, and as I was always ready to eat I didn't decline as the chips were poised at my lips.

However, when we got out of the bus at home the same young woman asked if I had some protection for her as she had started her period unexpectedly whilst at the market. We went into the office so I could find her some pads when I noticed her fingers were stained with dried blood, clearly from her menstrual problem. I was nearly sick, having been fed chips from this woman on the way home!

On another occasion we had some guests for a BBQ tea at the Mill. I was congratulating one of the young women on her delicious coleslaw she had made. We were all tucking in until she said she had enjoyed making it, apart from the fact that her fingernails had gone on her right hand whilst grating the carrots!

I couldn't understand or agree with new Government legislation in the nineties. It was deemed that some residents no longer had to pay for their care. The Government benefit system paid, leaving some residents with a large disposable income of around £100 a week. Nothing had to be paid out of this money other than their own personal needs. The system is so unfair. Some residents are left with £15 pocket money whilst others have a pocket full of money to spend as they wish. I'm not against a reasonable personal allowance being paid, but why can't a reasonable amount be given to everyone living in residential care? We were left with the 'rich and the poor'. The system changed when a court case was held and it was deemed that some residents were no longer responsible for their residential care fees. This also had a negative impact on Social Services budgets, because instead of resident and Social Services contribution to care, the whole expense was now the responsibility of Social Services. This meant that the budget was now only able to fund half the places as they were now paying the fees in full.

This account is from my eldest son Shane. Without the presence of the young people, children and pets our home would have been lacking the 'roundness' needed to call it our home. We have all gained a wealth of understanding and knowledge from each other.

The Mill – The Good, The Bad and The Horrendous

I get the impression from mum that looking back she felt that because of the demands of the business her kids were a little neglected. In my eyes I wouldn't have changed anything, and never felt that we were ever overlooked. Yes, there were times when Mum and Dave were not around, although no more than most parents who had successful careers. In fact as we lived next door to the home, one of them was normally on hand if we needed anything 24/7. We may just have had to share some of their attention with a resident trying to negotiate a loan for the next pack of fags.

Overall, I would say growing up at the Mill was an amazing experience and something I am really grateful for. I have a catalogue of interesting, unusual, sad and uplifting memories. Some of my favourites are below;

The Good:

The best part of living at the Mill for me was the laughs. I can't really remember many of the reasons why I laughed so much, but remember lots and lots of laughing and lots and lots of fun. It was the people who lived there who made it so entertaining, and there really were some amazing characters. Julian was probably one of the funniest people I have ever met, and seeing him make a sandwich with two tins of Hot Dog sausages, half a tub of mayo, four slices of bread and then demolishing it in two mouthfuls was amusing. There was also the time where he wanted to bet with me that he could woo one of the residents into bed even though she was in the process of preparing dinner for the whole house. Sure enough thirty minutes later Julian passed me in the living room hand in hand with the chef, giving me a wink and heading for one of the bedrooms.

I would definitely put football into my good experiences of the Mill. We used to have the best games of football, and I will never forget Peter's lazy left foot, Rodney in goal and Ricky down the wing, and we always had a gang of village mates who loved our games. We used to spend hours on the back field playing football, and these games were definitely helpful in my sports development at school. At school Rugby was not everyone's cup of tea, but I loved it and being chased by someone of the same age was never as scary as playing football with the 'ressies' like Dee, an 18 stone female with fag lit, determined for some recognition from anyone by doing anything she could to score a goal.

The Bad:

Smoking! I am certain I have seen more cigs smoked than anyone else in the world – and that was just from one resident!

Everyone seemed to smoke in the house and smoking seemed to be a massive part of the day-to-day dramas of the house. There seemed to be a number of different types;

The fagger who never had enough time to pull the fag away from the mouth, resulting in the length of ash hanging on for dear life to the butt, becoming too heavy and eventually hitting the floor.

The fagger who never had any, who spent all day scrounging, including from random people in the street who looked as though they may be kind enough to share a ciggy. Or even worse, going through ash trays retrieving butts to try and make a second hand cigarette.

There was also the fagger who tried to give up – EVERY DAY!

And the fagger who rationed their cigs to hourly smokes to stop smoking them all at once and then petitioning the staff to allow them to have their allowance early.

Smoking was definitely one of the worst memories for me, if not the worst.

The dreaded minibus! The bus was bad. Being a teenager stuck in a village was not always the most fun, and we often wanted to visit friends in town. I should be grateful that there was always someone from the house needing to go into town and we could always get a lift. However, this often meant going in the dreaded bus. Really it was silly to be embarrassed by getting a lift on the bus, but as a self-conscious teenager trying to be cool this came with <u>real</u> embarrassment!

Imagine being seen by school friends or a potential girlfriend who was unaware what your parents did for a living, seeing you getting off of a bus with a 20+ stone female crying because she no longer wanted to go into town, someone shouting at themselves at the top of their voice, JD smoking like it was the last fag on the planet and a white guy with dreadlocks trying to imitate Bob Marley and several passengers waiting to hop out at the first opportunity to smoke another fag which usually happened as I was getting dropped off.

Good memories and experiences definitely outweigh the bad memories which weren't that bad really, especially compared to the horrendous.

The Horrendous:

Dinner times at the Mill were sometimes revolting, and there were many occasions I remember eating there not being too glamorous. I remember the guy whose nose ran before he had managed to get out his handkerchief. The 'Big Fella' was great but ate so quickly that he looked as though when his plate of food was demolished he would continue to eat the plate, the cutlery and possibly even the person he was sitting next to.

There was the older lady who had terrible wind and had no problems releasing air (from both ends) no matter where she was, often resulting in a stench worse than bad eggs.

Retching could often be heard through the house and I am still mystified as to why this person didn't take a drop of liquid whilst taking medication? Every time the meds were dished out one particular resident would take the pills and then the retching would begin.

There were also the odd flashes of flesh which were unnecessarily shown, including the odd pair of boobs and sometimes even worse could be seen, including one chap's genitalia which seemed to have a terrible habit of falling out of his pyjamas.

There were horrid memories, but we had more fun times than not.

Finally, living at the Mill was really enjoyable and I feel privileged to have been able to have met so many interesting, weird and wonderful people. I enjoyed it so much that when I became an adult I even got involved in working a few shifts. On my very first, a very large lady decided to kill herself by jumping from her first floor bedroom window. On hearing a commotion I went to her room. The window was wide open and she shouted that she was going to jump. I took her by the arm and we span round in a frantic whirl, with me trying to manoeuvre her away from the window.

Meanwhile, Mum was 'taking afternoon tea' in another resident's room. Margaret had been a schoolteacher and this tea ritual was set for precisely 3pm – she wouldn't let you in if you were early. Hearing my cries for assistance, Mum excused and came to my rescue. Together, we were able to calm the large lady and get her to talk about her distress. Once the crisis had passed, Mum returned to Margaret's room to partake of tea from a china cup and eat cake!

That's how crazy, unpredictable life at The Mill could be, the crazy alongside the (almost) normal. I really enjoyed the work, which didn't feel like any other job I've done since.

LEE'S STORY:

Apparently my formative years were spent in an unusual community that I only ever regarded as being 'normal'. We moved to the Mill when I was seven years old so I had no reason to believe that my life was probably rather different to my peers. When the first residents arrived I just accepted them. They were always very pleasant to me and they were adults, so it wasn't for me to question their behaviour. I was never told why they lived with us, and I suppose I became very accepting of the occasional bizarre performance that was sometimes played out around me. More likely, I might be frustrated that this got in the way of something like playing football or going out on a trip. I can see in retrospect that perhaps these performances were brought on by anxiety about a forthcoming event. Looking back, I can see that my own non-judgemental attitude, though unwitting, was part of the very ethos of the Mill House. Whilst it was a far from 'normal' setting, there were expectations that everyone would partake equally in our small community.

I did get annoyed sometimes, particularly when one of the residents refused to dress appropriately and this messed up many a trip waiting for him to get ready and everyone got really bored waiting. There were endless hours of football with the residents and these were great fun. My friends from the village would come and join in and they too didn't give a second thought to the residents' behaviour, although when the residents were playing football their mental health issues seemed to pale into insignificance. I learnt that an important part of The Mill philosophy was that keeping people occupied distracted them from their problems.

I used to go away with Dave on the 'house holidays', usually camping in Derbyshire. These were great fun and to be honest it was like going away with your mates. Again the Millers were kept so busy walking, river crossing, climbing, swimming, horse-riding and going on scary night walks through the pitch black woods to the pub that eventually they would become so tired and all their problems lessened. Another of Mum's beliefs was that plenty of fresh air and exercise leads to a healthy mind. I lost count of the number of times residents were cajoled into something active and were doing it before they realized. Often you would see them taking the long walk from the front door to the minibus with a bewildered look on their faces that said 'Why am I doing this?'

There were also the camps at Maggie's farm. Mum always thought these were great fun and assumed we were also having a great time, but in reality they were set up for adults and for anyone who might be interested in music. I always felt threatened that Mum was going to get me on stage and get me to do something outrageous or 'hippified'. However, I do remember one occasion when my friend Dominic and I 'fixed' the raffle, winning a prize of Babycham (how uncool!) and getting rather drunk in the tent. I will always remember Wilm and Maggie with great fondness for their kindness and just being them.

One holiday took me, Mum, Maggie and several residents to Tunisia. Mum was about 35 weeks pregnant so the local men were very interested in her, feeling that she could be quite a prize. One of the residents with us was Julian Rostron; probably my favourite of all time. He was such a big and jolly chap with a fantastic belly laugh and a cool streak of mischievousness about him. He was such a lovely guy and wouldn't hurt a fly. The locals in the village called him 'Tyson' and he was really popular. Quite an achievement for a black guy in a Norfolk village in those days. Being with Julian for a week in Tunisia was just brilliant. Sadly his illness got the better of him in later years and he took his own life, knowing that life was never really going to be what he wanted for himself, but that's another story.

Looking back perhaps the strangest thing was my mother allowing me to be driven all over the country by various residents. They would take me to and from school or deliver me to friends' houses or wherever I needed to go. Generally it would all go fine, but on one occasion I remember Paul putting on a handbrake turn as he missed the turning. All great fun for a 13 year old. I think Mother just thought that somehow everything was going to be all right, so what was the worry. Dave often says that Mum lives in a 'pink fluffy world', but I guess it's all about being positive.

My younger brothers Jake and Charlie were also born whilst we lived at the Mill, but we eventually outgrew our cottage and had to move out. I guess they've had more of a normal upbringing than I did, but will have also missed out on having loads of 'playmates' (residents) at their beck and call. There was great excitement as Jake was born and I remember Mum letting one of the older female residents take him for long walks in his pram and she was gone for hours at a time. I think it's great to have so much trust in someone, and this was another part of The Mill House philosophy.

Gradually Mum and Dave acquired other houses and at one stage I was employed by them for a while. In truth I didn't particularly enjoy the work as somehow I'd been put in a totally different role and my relationship with the residents had changed by my being in a position of responsibility. Thus the fun had been taken out of what I knew previously, and regardless of my experience at the Mill House this was a step too far for me. Mum always had the endless positive opinion that you (that is me) must enjoy working with all these wonderful residents and I can't fault her infectious enthusiasm, but in all honesty it was great fun living with them but not my 'thing' to work with them. I think it was easier for me to accept them without question as a child rather than try to complicate matters by trying to accept and understand them as a young adult.

I still enjoy seeing the 'old timers' and they do stir up great memories and I thank them for that and also remember the ones that have sadly left us along the way. I guess I'll never know what 'normal' is but thanks for the experience.

Some professionals we worked with have their say;

Jan;

I am a community psychiatric nurse who visited the Mill many, many times to see and place clients there. Helen, Dave and their staff made it a welcoming, warm shelter for people with shattered lives who had often given up the hope of any happiness. The fragments were carefully put back together and given a shine, which lasted into their future. The Mill was a haven and was as good as it gets for those who need gently placing together.

Words from Valerie, a Social Worker from Peterborough:

I always thought Helen gave strong leadership to the staff team and down to earth common sense. I loved the way a resident could paint a wall frieze for the community and this was accepted without the home being 'on show'.

Alan Carr:

I met yourself and Dave in the mid 1980s, and visited you at the Mill fairly regularly for about five or six years. These were great times. There was a bunch of us who used to play music in your house once a week. We all worked in the NHS in the mental health field. We used to do occasional folk gigs at local pubs, and every year do a kind of concert for the gang at the Mill. By gang, I mean your clients. Also, from time to time, some of us would be involved in referring some of the clients we worked with in the NHS to the Mill, or offering them services while they were there. So that was the context within which I became familiar with the Mill and the sort of service yourself and Dave offered to your clients.

I've worked in mental health services in Canada, the UK and Ireland as a clinical psychologist. I'm also in contact with a large international network of professionals in the mental health field in my current job as Professor and Director of Clinical Psychology Training at University College Dublin. So I am familiar with the kinds of services that are available around the world for people recovering from mental health difficulties. I'm also involved at the moment in research on 'recovery' from psychological problems. My comments about the Mill are made with this stuff as a sort of backdrop.

The Mill was a remarkable place. You and Dave created a wonderfully warm, secure family-like environment within which your clients could live and work towards recovery. I admired the way you both in your different ways formed strong relationships with all your clients. You treated them all with respect, but never in a 'precious' way. You had a laugh with them, and didn't let them get away with behaving too bizarrely. You expected the best of them and in response much of the time they gave their best. You treated them as if they were capable of living a normal life. That was the thing about the Mill. It always looked to me like here was a great bunch of people living a normal life. You involved your clients in the day-to-day running of the household. Dave involved those who had an interest in the ongoing development of the property. You organized really enjoyable activities for all your clients. You were also always there for them. I was astonished at your continual personal generosity. It was obvious to any of us who visited the Mill how much you cared for your clients. The Mill and your clients never seemed to me like they were part of your job. They looked to me like they were a really important part of your life. I remember you developed the apartments too, so clients could move into them in their journey towards increasing independence. This was a great idea. You also worked in a very collaborative way with the various mental health professionals who were involved with your clients.

There is absolutely no comparison between the sort of service you offered, and the service provided by most of the 'mainstream' mental health residential facilities that I have come into contact with.

As they say here in Ireland Helen, 'If you could bottle what ever you did at the Mill and sell it to the Americans you would make a fortune'.

Gill Randall - Psychiatrist

It seems to me that the actual 'helping' of professional helping agencies these days is sometimes like an 'also-ran' amidst a sea of protocol and jargon – jargon like 'client centred service'.

But my memory of your Mill is that everything was about the people. About people just being people.

My time at the Mill – Simon Webb:

My association with the Mill and associated houses began in the summer of 1993 when I first went to an event at Maggie's Farm, meeting for the first time Dave, Helen and some of the residents, plus of course Maggie and Willem. A weekend to remember!! The following April in 1994 I began working part time at the Mill and so a new era of my life began in ways I could not have predicted.

Working over the next eighteen months or so was a learning experience in many different ways. I learned about the issues of mental health for the individual and society in general. If someone with mental health issues could wear a plaster cast then I'm sure those with reasonable mental health would be more sympathetic, because we can never tell when any of us might suffer from mental health issues.

Working in an environment like the Mill we can become aware that along with the real challenges that exist so do humour and good things. A trip to Somerset for a week's stay in a Youth Hostel in the autumn of 1994 is a concentrated reminder of that!

I was always intrigued to try and determine Dave and Helen's philosophy that underpinned the Mill environment. Even today I really can't say for certain. What I do think is that they cared deeply about all the residents (and the staff) and let those feelings and intuitions come into play – even against the dictates of the time. So I think the Mill environment grew organically and therefore flexibly, to enable them to support, provide a safe environment and to help those able to move back into general society.

So Dave and Helen, a job well done, and your 'retirement' is a loss to the Mental Health system in Norfolk.

Simon Webb Therapist: Dip Hyp., Master NLP Practitioner

In Conclusion

I hope you have enjoyed the rather unusual format of this book. I have been retired for three years now, but still keep in contact with many people who I worked with and alongside. My aim for the book was to cut the jargon and the stigma and allow you to see the colourful lives with the ups and downs that peoples' life journey takes them on.

It is the duty of all of us to both give and receive respect to and from each other without prejudice and to allow room for dignity, fun, laughter and love on the basis that we are all equal.

Helen

Thanks:

Catherine and Karen, my dear friends, have contributed so much to this book. It would have been such a struggle without them. Not only do they have inside information having lived and breathed it with me, they always knew where I was coming from. They have given me unconditional support and encouragement throughout – thank you both so much.
John, our old social worker student, another great help and support; I've enjoyed looking at your laptop screen with your old curry splatterings whilst we dismantled and evaluated my workings.

Thank you everybody who has contributed to this book. I am so grateful. Hopefully my grandchildren will have the opportunity to read this and realise how lucky their granny was in having such a privileged and interesting working life. Without the residents and staff I wouldn't have any tales of the Mill House and Community Support Homes to tell you, thank you.

I GONNA TELL YOU A STORY
OF A PLACE WHERE I'VE BEEN
AND IF YOU EVER GO THERE
YOU'LL THINK IT'S A SCREAM.
YOU'D NEVER FORGET THE PEOPLE YOU'D MET
COZ TO SEE THEM'S TO LOVE THEM
THAT'S THE REAL TREAT.

HELEN AND DAVE, THEY PICK 'EM EACH ONE
AND THAT'S WHERE I'VE BEEN
THE MILL HOUSE IN GAYTON.
THERE'S SOLLY AND ANDRE AND TERRY AS WELL.
A SMALL PERSON WITH HEART SO BIG AND
CONTRARY
AND THERE'S SALLY AND JOHN
AND OUR DEAR LADY MARY.

KAREN'S MOVED OUT TO A NICE LITTLE FLAT
CIGAR'S GONE WITH 'ER AND A BIG FLOPPY HAT
JASON HE HUGS YOU AND ASKS FOR A FAG.
ADY MY BUDDY, WE RAVE ON THE QUIET
COZ WHEN WE'RE TOGETHER FOLK THINK IT'S A RIOT
CATHERINE'S CHARACTER AS WITH ALL
THOSE WHO'RE THERE
WELL IT'S TOO BIG FOR WORDS
SO I JUST WOULDN'T DARE.

THAT WINDOW THEY SHUT IT
TRY THE STAFF, AS THEY MAY,
SAYS SOLLY "WE DON'T NEED NO
FRESH AIR TODAY".
TOM I KNEW YOU TWO YEARS AGO
WITH MY RED HAIR AND NOSE PIERCED,
AND FAG ON THE GO
JULIA MY MATIE, SO GENTLE, SO NEW
YOU'VE MADE THAT FIRST STEP
THAT YOU NEEDED TO.
IAN I SMILE WHEN I THINK OF YOUR FACE

YOUR SPECIAL LITTLE LAUGH
ALWAYS FILLS UP A SPACE.

BEFORE I JUST STAYED IN AND
TALKED OF MY PROBLEMS,
BUT NOW I HAVE HEALTH
AND I'M LIVING SOLUTIONS.
THE MILL, IT'S SPECIAL
AND THE PEOPLE THEY CARE,
EVEN THOUGH YEARS HAVE PASSED
WITH THE THOUGHT 'LIFE'S UNFAIR'.

NOW IS YOUR TIME,
COME ON BANDAGE THOSE WOUNDS
THERE'S A FUTURE OUT THERE
FOR YOU IF YOU CHOOSE.

SO TO ALL MILLERS BE THIS MESSAGE OF FATE,
NO MATTER WHO YOU ARE, IT'S NEVER TOO LATE.

Written by Sarah Pye.

Lightning Source UK Ltd.
Milton Keynes UK
UKOW050707170212

187478UK00001B/10/P